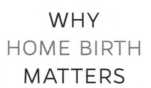

WHY
HOME BIRTH
MATTERS

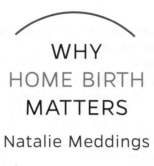

WHY
HOME BIRTH
MATTERS

Natalie Meddings

Why Home Birth Matters (Pinter & Martin Why It Matters 11)

First published by Pinter & Martin Ltd 2018

©2018 Natalie Meddings

Natalie Meddings has asserted her moral right to be identified as the author of this work in accordance with the Copyright, Designs and Patents Act of 1988.

ISBN 978-1-78066-555-9

Also available as an ebook

Pinter & Martin Why It Matters ISSN 2056-8657
Series editor: Susan Last
Index: Helen Bilton
Cover Design: Blok Graphic, London
Cover illustration: Sam Kalda
Proofreader: Debbie Kennett

British Library Cataloguing-in-Publication Data

A catalogue record for this book is available from the British Library.

Set in Minion

Printed and bound in the UK by Ashford Colour Press Ltd, Gosport, Hampshire

This book has been printed on paper that is sourced and harvested from sustainable forests and is FSC accredited.

Pinter & Martin Ltd
6 Effra Parade
London SW2 1PS
pinterandmartin.com

Contents

Contents

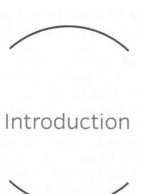

Introduction

This is a book about having babies at home. What it means. Why it works. How it feels. I'm eager to jump right in – to show and share some extraordinary things. They will stir you, surprise you and, in all probability, change your life. But first, there's something we need to take care of.

Say the word 'home' and see what it summons. Your kitchen and its kettle? Or where you sit in the evening to watch a film? Maybe a sigh, your body's way of explaining it – registering the comfort of a key in the door.

Now try the word 'birth'. It grabs and distils something doesn't it? There's a bit of uncertainty, maybe. But a *baby*. A beginning. A word that describes where being alive starts.

And then try 'home birth'. Combined, those two tiny words feel instantly complicated. Incongruent. Whether a person is open to and opting for a home birth, or is opposed to it and convinced that the concept is insane, it can be a burdened term.

'Home birth' is so tied to kneejerk notions of what makes

birth safe, of what is 'normal', and with there being a 'type' of person that takes this path, that thinking about it is often already done – *by someone else* – which makes it impossible for women to freely inform themselves *for* themselves and consider having a baby at home in a balanced way.

The term home birth has us either over-investing and staking our all on it, or rejecting it out of hand. My feeling is that we should put all this aside, and clarify what having a baby at home involves by examining the facts. Is it safe? Is it manageable? How is labour served by a home setting? What are the benefits of meeting your new baby in your own space?

I was pregnant with my second child when I first noticed how loaded the term 'home birth' can be. My first baby had been born in a free-standing birth centre in north London, and as all had gone well, my plan was to do everything the same again. I remember someone suggesting a home birth and immediately dismissing it. My mind whirled with what-ifs, don't-tempt-fates, and, more nagging than either, an insistent voice whispering, 'you're not the type'.

And then I got a doula. 'Why don't you see how you go?' she said. 'If you book a midwife to come to your home, you can see how you feel and decide then. Why shut down your options?'

She'd waved a wand. In a single puff, my reservations went up in smoke. My thinking cleared. Put like that, I could see how giving birth at home didn't have to be a fixed decision, some big, no-going-back test. It was a flexible, open-ended, common-sense arrangement, highly suited to my situation – a healthy woman, enjoying a healthy pregnancy, where the likeliest outcome was a straightforward birth.

Being able to wait and see meant there was less to think about. On the day itself, I could tune into the here-and-now without distraction, and respond directly to each feeling without taking stock of who or what was around me. In my own, private uninterrupted space, my body's instructions were as decisive and clear as any involuntary physical urge, and so I followed them – leaning forward on my bed and closing my eyes; resting on the floor beside my ironing board. Descending the stairs, one step, one contraction at a time, until I reached the warm water of my birth pool at the bottom, got in and gave birth to my new baby girl. It was the surest thing my body had ever done.

It's hard to imagine birth being easy. It may be only decades that women have been giving birth in managed, medicalised environments as a matter of routine. But the steep rise in emergency outcomes and drawn-out, exhausting labours that has accompanied this particular approach, and which we hear about and see in the media, has left a deep dent in our confidence.

Besides this, new mothers now were born to a generation of mothers who themselves had no memory of or cultural reference for birth taking place outside of a hospital. Meaning birth as something to manage and endure now feels like a necessary reality. A fact of life.

But it's not a fact of life. And women haven't always felt that way. In the first half of the 20th century women gave birth to their babies at home in large numbers – the vast majority successfully and most of them more easily than we do today.

There was a chain of confidence, a shared understanding of what to expect and what would be needed. And reinforcing both was the uncomplicated, routine practice whereby a midwife came to the house when you were in labour.

There was none of the pressure of a home birth 'plan'. No unnecessary decision-making to distract. A healthy woman saw birth as a normal function of the body and contractions a necessary by-product of that. So when labour unfolded normally, as for most it did, she stayed put, reassured and safely supported by her skilled and attentive midwife.

On the rare occasion that birth didn't follow a straightforward path, a GP would be called or she'd go to hospital.

Today, knowledgeable woman-to-woman support is rare; anxiety and feelings of helplessness are common; there is little or no understanding of what to expect or what is needed and many mothers feel scared and unqualified, accepting their 'lot' with a kind of dazed, incurious patience. So, unsurprisingly, when a well-meaning midwife moots to a mother the possibility of having her baby at home, the idea feels wildly way-off. Unthinkable.

There's a kind of unquestioning indifference to this standard reaction. Why women make the decisions they do around birth at home, and birth generally, are left unexplored – 'choice' having become something of an unchallengeable sacred cow.

But as so much decision-making is rooted in and shaped by outsized fear, poor understanding, scare stories, distorting media coverage and a lack of birth education, isn't what's being made a *choiceless* choice? Isn't it the case, as midwife of 30 years Sheena Byrom suggests, that women 'don't know what they don't know'?

Why Home Birth Matters is a solution. It's a storehouse of relevant, useful, accurate information, built on biology, experience and ordinary women's wisdom. And its aim is to ensure that you *do* know.

Giving birth is generally very safe for both you and your baby, wherever you choose to give birth, according to the gold-standard National Institute for Clinical Excellence (NICE) guidelines. And the years I've spent accompanying women through birth as a doula – hundreds of them at home

– mean I can vouch for that. Each birth journey has added to my own 'birth' journey, helping me to learn new pearls each time. Ways to soothe, labour's reassuringly predictable rhythms, what can interrupt and alter a birth's course. And, most importantly, the many ways a woman can be protected from disturbance and her labour helped to happen.

You'll find it all gathered here. From the first chapters, which help you work through the decision of having a baby at home, to more practical guidance, like how it can bring out the best in your body, pacing yourself and coping.

Supporting women in birth has given me the know-how that fills this book. But the bedrock beneath it was being blessed with the best of teachers: Janet Balaskas, founder of the active birth movement, the guardian of normal birth; obstetrician Michel Odent; some magical midwives who know who they are and, finally, the mother-doula, Liliana Lammers, whose warm, clever hands helped me have my babies. They showed me true north – the power of normal birth when normal birth has what it needs.

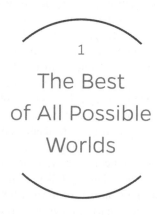

1

The Best
of All Possible
Worlds

It's easy to find reasons *not* to have a baby at home. In the opinion of our culture-at-large, there are plenty of them. Birth is too dangerous. Too painful. Too unpredictable. Even too messy.

As few of us get round to asking where all these 'toos' have come from, there this thinking sits – layers of sediment built on stories heard, assumptions made and terrifying television portrayals that have about as much to do with real birth as porn does with real sex.

So let's do something. Let's hose the mud away. You wouldn't base other life-defining decisions on hand-me-down opinion. Or scary stories. Or what the papers say. If having a baby at home is to be included as a serious choice, the first step is to wash off all the hearsay – about birth being hugely painful or massively risky – and start with the facts.

Most people assume that hospital is the safest place to have a baby. But this is mostly based on the fact that everyone else is having their baby in hospital – a setting which will see four in ten women having a caesarean or instrumental delivery and where 86% of women end up being medically managed on an obstetric ward. (NHS Maternity Statistics 2016/17, National Maternity Review: Better Births)

Given that most women *want* a normal birth* without intervention (The National Maternity Review Better Births research shows that only 25% of women would choose to give birth on a medical labour ward) and that the evidence points to there being a low chance of that happening in hospital, it's important to understand why having a baby at home is a viable, safe alternative. In fact, in the context of good standards of health and high-quality maternity care, it might even provide the best of all possible worlds.

The turning point for us was a course we attended, where we found out what happens when you give birth and what the body needs for it to happen easily. Just hearing the facts made me realise that appalling examples of childbirth on telly like One Born Every Minute *have a lot to answer for, showing terrified women, being pumped full of drugs, lying on their backs as their partners look on helplessly.*

Once I learned how labour worked and what helped it happen, I understood how it didn't have to be that way. We live six floors up and I was already feeling anxious about going into labour during rush hour, getting out of the building into a taxi. It just didn't feel right at any point and finally, I simply asked myself, 'Where do I feel most safe?' The answer was my home.

---

* The Association for Improvements in Maternity Services (AIMS) has defined normal birth as 'a physiological birth where the baby is delivered vaginally following a labour which has not been altered by technological interventions'.

Hospital never appealed to me instinctively, but educating myself about childbirth confirmed that there were good reasons for my instincts. There were no downsides to having my baby at home at all. The only way it would have been a problem is if we had not done any preparation beforehand. But we made sure we properly educated ourselves. When the midwife arrived about an hour and a half before Nancy was born, I thought she would want to do an internal exam. Instead she simply said, very quietly and calmly, 'It's OK, I know how far along you are'. She was so skilled at reading my body, and that gave me confidence, to trust and follow my body too.

Kate

Labour is a need. Though it's more commonly regarded as a process, what drives that process is physical necessity – that the mature baby now sustains itself, is an issue of survival for you both. Re-understanding birth like this, as something your body and baby are physically and instinctively *compelled* to do, makes it easier to see birth for what it is – a hugely reliable physical function.

Women have been successfully giving birth with little or no intervention for many thousands of years because their bodies are designed to do so. The varying caesarean rates of different countries (Turkey 50%; Sweden 16%), a 2010 World Health Organization report estimating that 6.2 million unnecessary caesarean sections were performed every year, and even the varying intervention rates from one local hospital to another (see Birthchoice UK), all indicate that the incidence of women requiring aid or rescue is less to do with the reliability of birth and more to do with the health system and prevailing culture in a particular country or area.

'The idea that birth should be efficient has its roots in the 17th century when men used science to redefine birth (Donnison 1988)', writes Dr Rachel Reed, author of online blog midwifethinking.com. 'The body was conceptualised as a machine and birth became a process with stages, measurements, timelines, mechanisms etc. This is still reflected in current textbooks, knowledge and practice'.

This mechanistic view of birth and the medical control that accompanied it became so dominant in the late 20th century that most of us are now unaware that the ability to birth is inbuilt. The process of labour is completely involuntary, like breathing, or sleep. Did you know that there are cases where women have given birth vaginally while in a coma?

These days it's hard to believe our bodies instinctively know what they're doing. Women feel tasked with '*giving* birth', most believing that the successful arrival of their child is dependent on their own individual physical capacity and performance – whether or not they have the right-sized pelvis, a cervix that will dilate, a pain threshold that's high enough, or simply adequate strength and fitness.

From an evolutionary perspective, it's obvious that the survival of the human race wouldn't base itself on a lottery – randomly gambling person to person, pelvis to pelvis, in the hope of success.

The ability to birth is hardwired into our DNA. Labour is an automatic universal function of human physiology. But understanding of this is sketchy and our trust in it – a key component for allowing the whole thing to happen in the first place – has almost entirely disappeared.

Control of the birth process has of course brought benefits – greater safety and improved outcomes for high-risk pregnancies and in cases of legitimate emergency. But routine over-control of all pregnancies, at the expense of women being given what they need to let labour happen, has compromised natural competence. The mass-persuading of women that management by experts is imperative if labour is to happen at all, let alone safely, has robbed women of the one thing they do need: confidence.

One hundred years ago, when around 90% of babies were born at home, relying solely on this physical template wasn't enough. Though there was still a view that 'pregnancy and childbirth is a natural physiological event... and departures from the normal occur in a small proportion of cases', there were too many other factors influencing outcomes, like poverty, poor health and insanitary conditions. Even when the Notification of Birth Acts of 1907 and 1915 gave grants to local authorities in order to provide antenatal visits to women in their homes, assessment of pregnant women's health would have been rudimentary. For example, a mother going into labour with a pelvis distorted by rickets (a condition caused by malnutrition) would have easily been missed.

Just over half a century later, the complete opposite was the case. R.D. Laing's disturbing 1978 film depicting the degrading conveyor-belt practices of hospital birth that continued into the 1980s showed the inevitable result of attempts to eliminate all risk: mothers trussed in stirrups, sedated and tethered to machines, 'and chemicals used routinely to control the whole course, tempo and rhythm of uterine contractions'. Some safety practices of the period even *increased* danger, with research eventually confirming that the single consistent consequence of routine continuous electronic foetal monitoring (CTG) was an increased need for caesarean section.

Today, things are different. Lessons have been learned. As a result of the awareness-raising efforts of birth activists like Sheila Kitzinger, Janet Balaskas, Ina May Gaskin and obstetrican Michel Odent, the more industrial extremes of maternity care have been moderated and normal birth physiology is now acknowledged and, to a point, provided for.

At the other end of the scale, a pregnant woman no longer has to take her chances. As well as there being a greater standard of health generally, we now enjoy the benefit of free pregnancy assessment and continuous midwife care throughout pregnancy, meaning that a full-term pregnant woman will have a clear and accurate picture of both her own and her baby's wellbeing. Add in that skilled midwife care is available throughout labour and high-quality medical backup is there if required, and we find ourselves in a historically unique situation.

Birth has never been safer.

This signals an opportunity – we can now place some fitting faith in our own fit-for-purpose female biology. We don't routinely presume other organs or physical functions are going to fail. We justifiably run our lives on the basis of the likeliest outcome – that our lungs or heart, for example, will do their job. But as 98% of women choose to have their baby in a maternity care setting, we clearly don't invest the same trust in our uterus.

Despite all the evidence to the contrary, expectant mothers – especially first-time mothers – assume that problems in birth are likely. And it is this misbelief – that a first birth entails many more variables and unknowns than subsequent births – that causes most first-time mothers to dismiss birth at home out of hand.

But what is this based on? Haphazard outcomes aren't what the statistics show. On the contrary, report after report has confirmed that for a healthy woman experiencing an uncomplicated pregnancy, a straightforward birth is by far the likeliest outcome. Medical help is only likely to be required in a small minority of cases, meaning routine hospital care for all is an inappropriate and heavy-handed insurance policy.

So many people told me I was mad to be having my first child at home. Lots of them told me to expect a hospital transfer. Every time it came up, I'd get a raised eyebrow, and that made me angry, because it was opinion based on ignorance.

There's this assumption that hospital is where you're safe – and that if you're having a baby at home, you're being irresponsible and taking a big risk. Not one of the people who told me I was mad had the first idea about the statistics, or how labour works, or what I would actually need physically to give birth easily. And yet still people feel able to have that opinion, and do all they can to influence yours. It's amazing really, as how acceptable would women find being patronised and controlled in other areas of their life?

Everyone is brainwashed into thinking that childbirth is a risky business. Even when I do tell people I had my baby at home, almost always I get same the same reply; 'It's lucky nothing went wrong'. No questions, no enquiry. In fact, some things did go 'wrong'. But that's another myth – the notion of safety being either/or. That hospital is where there's a solution, and at home you're high and dry. I'd much prefer having the skilled, exclusive attention of one midwife, attending me and me only, than have to share a midwife on a labour ward, who may be distracted or tired from having to juggle the needs of several women. When my midwife had to help me, it was peaceful. There was no panic – she simply dealt with the issue calmly and I didn't know about anything until my daughter was safe in my arms.

Kate

Evidence that hospital might not be the safest place to give birth began to gather in the 1980s, when research statistician Marjorie Tew's analysis of maternity data made some surprising discoveries. Her findings, which were published in the *Journal of the Royal College of General Practitioners*, demonstrated that hospital was only of benefit to women at very high risk of complications, and that for low-risk women the risks of having a baby in a consultant unit were higher than having a planned birth at home.

Changing Childbirth, the landmark 1993 report that further identified how increased medicalisation and standardisation of maternity care reduced the chances of a normal birth outcome, went on to officially reverse the policy that hospital was the safest place to give birth, and the recent 2016 Cochrane Review on Maternity Care and the Department of Health's Birthplace in England Research Programme have reached the same conclusions. These are that:

1. Giving birth is generally very safe.
2. Midwife-led care results in a higher chance of a spontaneous vaginal birth.

The Birthplace study (2011) also found that for first-time mothers giving birth at home there was only a slight increase in risk as compared to those giving birth in hospital, and that for second-time mothers, the risks were actually higher in hospital.

It was a male colleague asking me where I was going to have my baby that first got me to consider my options properly. I had automatically opted for hospital as it hadn't even occurred to me there was another choice. He was normally such an unemotional man – the head of maths at the school I worked at – so I was taken aback by how unexpectedly passionate and persuasive he was about it.

As soon as I started to research it I knew I wanted to give it a try – two dedicated midwives in my own home with no transfer to hospital stress. I was 10 minutes from my local hospital, so had a good safety net. It was a no-brainer, and on the day itself it seemed the most natural, normal thing to do in all the world – to welcome our baby into our home. And it would have felt entirely unnatural, strange even, to opt for a setting that was sterile, alien, noisy and unknown. There was no fuss, no negotiation, no second-guessing, no distractions. I was able to listen to what my body was telling me and go with it. I could be completely present for the most amazing experience of my life – and then all be tucked up together in bed, me, my husband and my baby, just a few hours later.

Helen

I was a journalist before training as a doula, and one day I got sent to interview a teenage girl who'd given birth secretly in her bedroom on Christmas day. When things began, she'd paced her room while her parents basted potatoes and sipped sherry in the kitchen below.

As her contractions intensified, she hung from the window-frame, where she found the icy, cold air soothing to breathe. She felt how sitting on the toilet brought the best relief when she started to feel pressure in her back and bottom, got on all fours when that felt even better, and shortly after gave birth to her baby girl on a towel she'd laid out on the floor. I was fascinated. At the time, I thought birth was something quite frightening, so to see how unfazed and physically self-assured this girl had been was amazing to me. She'd done no reading, attended no classes – and though she'd been anxious about her parents' reaction to the baby, when it came to the birth itself, she'd been sanguine: her body had made and grown her baby. It was common sense to her that her body had a plan for getting it out.

Many would claim that this girl's quick and straightforward birth was because she was young. But that's just one part of it. When a woman is in safe, quiet, uninterrupted surroundings, the birth process is often efficient in this way, as the very high normal birth rate in the 1940s and 50s, a time when large numbers of women were having their babies at home, confirms.

Midwives and doulas who've spent years supporting women at home will tell you the same. When there is no disorienting unfamiliarity; no management of your behaviour; no disruptive changes in atmosphere and no disturbing sounds or activity, something wonderful happens – something so obviously helpful it's amazing it's been forgotten for so long.

The mother works around the birth. Instead of the birth having to work around everything else – baby and body having to fit in with prescribed timeframes, or wrap themselves around a fixed setting or medical agenda – the birth leads the way. Undistracted, the mother can concentrate on her body's cues and has full and uninhibited opportunity to express her birthing instinct.

At home, in my own private, protected space, my body became a force of nature – a powerful, muscular force of nature. All I had to do was get out of the way and let it get on with the job. It's so simple if you think about it. We give our body the conditions it needs to help other physical processes, like privacy and a vertical receptacle for going to the loo; darkness and safety for going to sleep.

And yet we wonder why giving birth, a process a thousand times more sensitive, becomes so hard to do in a busy, brightly-lit public institution where the environment is transactional and ever-changing, full of variables and uncertainty.

Imagine trying to sleep in an airport departure lounge, seated upright, surrounded by strangers, constantly checking the monitor for your flight. Being in labour in hospital feels the same. I did it that way the first time, and never again. You may get a private room in hospital, but a small space has its limits. There's only so much bouncing on a ball you can do. In your own home, there are no restrictions, no decisions – you are free. And when you're free, you can let go.

Sarah

Women's lives have altered overwhelmingly for the better in the last century, change having brought equality in education, career opportunity, and the opening up of choice and ordinary freedom on every level. Except in childbirth. Ironically, it's here, in exclusively female territory, that women can feel weak and ill-equipped.

If workplace conditions were holding us back in the same way, we would do something about it. We'd work out what was hampering us, and take reasoned, constructive steps to give ourselves the best chance to fulfil our potential. So why not do the same with birth?

Having a baby at home won't be the right decision for everyone. But it will be the right decision for many, given that the requirements for a simple labour are universal. At home, in your own safe, private, familiar territory, labour can progress more easily. There is no need to interrupt labour to go into hospital and there's a much greater feeling of all-round control. You can choose who you want present at the birth and there is a high chance that you will be looked after by a midwife you'll have met before or know well. You get to find your own way, in your own way. What more could you want?

For me, a home birth was absolutely the best of all possible worlds. It was my own space. I had all my own comforts, like blankets, pillows, my own food and of course, the loo. When having surges while on the toilet, it was my bathroom I was in; my floor I was kneeling on. I had my husband with me, but also my mum. She was just downstairs, popping up every now and then with a hug. She was there for my husband and for me. It wouldn't have been like that in hospital. At home she was present the whole time.

Besides all this, my midwife was the same midwife I had seen through pregnancy, which was amazing. She was experienced, calm and fully focused on me and my labour. She also faded into the background, again not something that would have happened in hospital, and that meant I could relax. There is a lot of negativity around first-time mums and home births. But we made our decision looking at facts. We learned that, when things go wrong, it is extremely rare for that to happen quickly. There is a lead up and warnings that a midwife is trained to watch for and get me to hospital if needs be. I had no reservations once I knew that. I felt completely reassured.

Jane

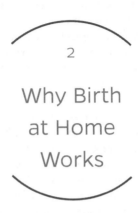

2

Why Birth at Home Works

In your own home, your body has exactly what it needs to labour with ease. Comfort. Control. Freedom. Time. Trust. In your own environment, these ingredients are in plentiful, natural supply and, when brought together, act as a catalyst – helping the birth to happen.

Birth at home becomes an unhurried happening – unfolding in your own comfortable time, on your own uninhibited terms.

What drives birth?

Birth is run by the hypothalamus – the primitive bit of the brain that's entrusted with the non-negotiable activities of the body, things that have to be taken care of like hunger, temperature control, sleep – and, just as vitally, childbirth.

While the neocortex responds moment-to-moment, thinking, reasoning and evaluating as it goes, the body needs the super-reliable hypothalamus to act as a hard drive, to run the automatic processes that keep us alive. And that includes labour. The successful arrival and survival of a new baby isn't down to the individual mother. It is an involuntary biological process that your body will get on and do – because it's hardwired to.

How does it begin?

Towards the end of pregnancy, the weight of your baby draws them down into the pelvis and onto the cervix. The deeper your baby descends, the more pressure their head applies and this is the signal for the hypothalamus to start oxytocin production. It messages the pituitary gland to begin releasing this vital birth hormone, which is what sets the muscles of the uterus contracting. Contractions cause the womb's muscle fibres to become more and more tightly knit, drawing the neck of the womb up and over your baby's head.

Contractions are usually spaced and uncoordinated at first, as their aim at this stage is just to get things ready.

The weave of the womb gathers with each wave and, as the available space decreases, the baby is forced to head for where there's more room – the soft, stretchy and now yielding cervix.

Throughout pregnancy, the cervix is long and thick and the opening – the os – firmly closed. But when you are full-term, an increase in prostaglandins helps to dissolve its soft tissue, making the cervix thin and stretchy. With the baby weighing ever more heavily, the cervix now starts to let go, giving and opening in response to the baby's nudging crown.

Labour is underway

A feedback loop is established. The more the baby presses, the more messages the brain receives to release oxytocin. Increased oxytocin leads to stronger and more frequent contractions, which lead to even more pressing by the baby... and on it goes, a cumulative, pace-gathering, exquisitely levered series of muscular decisions that draw and drive the baby down and through the pelvis.

Imagine pulling on a polo-neck jumper. At first, you have to wiggle your head and tug on the jumper to get the neck to give over the top of your head. But once it's midway, as far as your ears, it hits a tipping point – and your head slides easily through. This is how dilation works. The baby's head moves through the cervix in the same way.

Helping the baby to do this is the mother's mobile, pliable, purpose-built pelvis. Composed of several moving bones and, in pregnancy, ligaments that have been softened by the hormone relaxin, the pelvis is designed to accommodate and adapt around the baby's descending head.

Hips spread, sacrum and tailbone release and the internal mould of the pelvis encourages the baby to tuck their chin ever closer to their chest, to optimise a diameter-precise dive through the pelvic outlet.

A labouring mother will swing and sway her hips; rock and tip her bottom, lean forward, lift a leg or lie on her side – spontaneously and unthinkingly moving and positioning her body in a way that enlists gravity, makes room in her pelvis and helps her baby to be born.

The lower her baby goes, the more oxytocin is released. Once labour is established, and contractions very powerful, this hormone, which is labour's fuel, leads her deeper into her automatic self, helping her to let go of thinking, self-awareness and control, and to hand over to the involuntary pull of the feelings her body is producing.

There is terrific, conductive power to advanced labour. Like a current, the labour surges through the body, driving the process forward with powerful charge and rhythm, so that the baby can be born.

Like sleep, established labour feels like an irresistible urge

– something you've no choice over. And as with sleep too, the mother will instinctively seek out a private, protected unstimulating space so that the urge won't be suppressed.

She won't want to think, act or be 'in charge' of herself. She needs an environment so safe and undemanding that no neocortical alertness is required at all and the hypothalamus can take over and drive the birth to a safe conclusion.

The baby arrives

With the sleeve of the cervix cleanly over and behind their head, the baby can start moving down into the birth canal. With no cervix to stimulate, contractions can slow and space and this gives the mother a natural rest. She will have already felt a growing heaviness in her lower back and bottom as labour has been progressing; that feeling now intensifies as the baby's head moves past the rectum and starts pressing heavily on the pelvic floor, perineum and anus, stretching and opening everything up.

Soaring oxytocin levels have reduced self-consciousness, so that, relaxed and uninhibited, she instinctively gives way to the urgent sensation of her body expelling the baby.

Interiorly, this is felt as extreme pressure, which she has no choice but to join in with, culminating in an involuntary urge to bear down.

The baby's head is born. The force of contractions, as well as the internal shape of the pelvis, helps the baby to rotate on to its side a final time, to give space for the shoulders, which release one after the other, followed by the whole body.

Home is where the body works

Ordinarily, I avoid giving anatomy lessons. I don't believe it helps women much, to analyse their insides or be shown diagrams of labour's stages. We don't need an intellectual grasp of how to sleep in order to sleep and birth is no different. My mum didn't know what a cervix was. My nanna wouldn't have even known what a vagina was. But they both gave birth without difficulty, as most women did and do when they trust the process and let their body get on with it.

So the reason for the nuts and bolts detail above is to get you thinking – about how intricate and physiologically well-organised birth is. And then to consider, with care, how you are going to provide for that – what your body is going to *need* if it's to function optimally and give birth without complication.

The current cultural consensus continues to convince us that hospital is an appropriate place to birth. But is it the best place biologically?

The birth process is involuntary, but it is sensitive. Labour is automatic, but it is easily disturbed.

It's true that your body is fully equipped and capable of giving birth normally. But it works on the basis that you're going to give it the right conditions: the fullest possibility of the pelvis being free; total lack of disturbance, so that you can switch off and relax; and an atmosphere that helps oxytocin to release.

'Women now cannot release the hormone they are supposed to be releasing for giving birth – oxytocin,' says obstetrician Michel Odent. 'We have completely forgotten what the basic needs of a labouring woman are – the things that help that hormone to release. Privacy, feeling safe and not feeling observed.'

Hospital settings and routine maternity care mostly disregard these physiological needs – from brightly-lit reception areas and sensor-lit loos, to timeframes for labour and dilation scores.

Whether you're going to a labour ward or a birth centre,

both journey and arrival will require you to be alert, to engage with people you've never met and a busy, brightly-lit place you don't know, and, given maternity care admission criteria, all this while you're in active labour.

Your room is a public, unfamiliar space, with a smell and feel you don't know. Like any institution, a hospital setting requires a level of compliance and control to function smoothly – so you will feel a need to communicate and cooperate. You are limited to one room; your partner has one chair, and there will be one pillow. You will likely be sharing your midwife with other mothers and when her shift is over, a new person will take over.

Consider how easy it would be to perform other natural functions if they were being managed in this way – *trying* to sleep or having to consciously *think* your way to an orgasm, an act of physical release equally driven by the hormone oxytocin.

We wouldn't attempt to doze off in the aisle of a noisy supermarket. Or live in a house without a toilet. And yet we expect to give birth – an involuntary act of the exact same sort – in an environment that doesn't provide for it. On our backs usually, despite birth being a vertical, gravity-aided activity. And on display, when birth is dependent on unthinking disinhibition.

It's no wonder 'failure to progress' is so frequently the reason for obstetric assistance. Unsuitable, stimulating conditions act like a stress-test on the labour process, slowing and even halting physiological flow.

It is of course possible to adapt hospital rooms and make them comfortable – for lights to be lowered and soft stuff provided. And you can use earplugs, shawls and relaxation downloads to block distractions and help you settle in. And if you do need to go to hospital at any point, you can employ all these methods to help you feel more comfortable, which in turn will help your body to birth your baby. But just reflect for a moment on the idea that the very things you need – peace, quiet, privacy and freedom, and all your familiar and favourite things – are all available to you, freely and unrestrictedly, at home.

Hospital-based birth has brought some improvements to how babies are born, the greatest being highly-skilled medical support in cases of legitimate emergency. It's also true that some women will only feel safe in hospital – making it the right choice for them.

But for a far greater number of women, who have neither complex issues in pregnancy, nor high levels of anxiety, a medicalised setting can make things more complicated, and it will be their own home that gives them what they need.

At home, you can get comfortable without thinking. Find a safe, soft, enclosing space, without requesting it. Your midwife may be someone you've got to know, and your partner can relax and be himself.

A further benefit of not having to manage yourself is the way it helps with coping, by altering the experience and perception of contractions. Instead of pain being the primary focus, the intensifying waves of pressure that move a birth forward are felt for what they are – necessary and normal. There's no need to time them, or to plot progress: labour is marked out by your feeling of it.

One aim of standardising maternity care and presenting it as a linear process was to increase certainty and predictability. In practice, the opposite has happened.

Today labour lengths and outcomes vary hugely, but giving birth hasn't always been a lottery in that way – nor mothers' bodies such a mystery to them. And that's apparent when women birth at home. Female physiology has its fullest chance to function, the mother follows the path her body carves – and labour makes sense.

I was only half way through my pregnancy but I'd noticed a growing anxiety in me about birth. At first I thought it was about the process itself – the pain, the unpredictability – and even considered booking for an elective caesarean. I thought that way, the worry would be taken away and I'd feel in control. But then I saw a film where the obstetrician Michel Odent explains the way cultural interference has taken away women's power to give birth. That it was the way we 'do' birth now that makes it so nerve-wracking. It was like a switch had flicked.

I now knew what I wanted because I knew what I needed. 'We cannot help a mother to give birth', he said, 'it's an involuntary process and all we can do is protect her from disturbance, from inhibitory factors'. It made so much sense. No light, no language, no sense of being observed – even though I'd not done it before, I could feel instinctively how important that would be. How the only way I could ensure it was staying at home. I've got a plan now. I've booked a doula, I'm having midwife appointments from my local community team and when I'm in labour, they'll come to me in my own home. Now I can sleep well – having this plan has helped me to relax.

Helen

A doula's story...

Sam had been having very powerful contractions at home and not much change for some time... but that didn't matter as she hadn't had a vaginal examination so there was no clock to worry about. Free of an arbitrary timeframe, there was no 'place' she was supposed to have got to. Things had ramped up when her midwife had left after dropping by earlier. And now, on heading for the toilet, she felt things deepen again. With the door closed, and the possibility of completely letting go, she felt the urge to bear down. Hearing her noises change, her midwife, who'd been back a while but had stayed in the background, put her head round the door, helped Sam to lean forward and, with a couple of surges, her baby was born. Physiology may be a magical thing to behold – but there is nothing unexpected about it. It's pure biology, hard science. Darkness and privacy (or at least not feeling observed) will propel a labour forward like nothing else. And yet still people are surprised when a baby is born easily in such conditions.

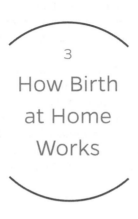

3

How Birth at Home Works

Giving birth at home makes biological sense. It also makes emotional sense, as it provides the highest chance of a straightforward birth, which in turn brings the benefits of optimal wellbeing and bonding for you and your baby. Now for the practical part – what you need to do to help your home birth to happen.

What follows is a lot of information, but the devil is in the detail. As well as it being helpful to know the nuts and bolts of how having a baby at home works, it's necessary to examine how midwife care at home currently stands up as a service.

Home birth needs to be a reliable, accessible, well-signposted option for women across the UK, and in various sorts of circumstances, if the service is to be available to and used by women as standard.

The first step

Whether you are mildly curious, actively interested or entirely certain you want to stay at home to have your baby, the first step is to get clear on how it all works – from how to book midwife care at home, to what that care will involve, in pregnancy, for the birth, and right after you've had your baby.

You will have been informed about your place of birth choices at your booking-in appointment. It should have been explained to you that home is a safe place to have your baby and that current clinical evidence confirms that midwife-led care at home is a positive and very safe option.

If this conversation didn't happen, you can ask the midwife about it at your next appointment, as NICE guidelines state that pregnant women should be provided with complete information on all their options for maternity care and place of birth.

Some people start considering staying at home to have

Two concerns women often have about home birth are:

'I'm worried about my neighbours and the noise'.
'I've got a small, rented flat. What about all the mess?'

Let's clear these stumbling blocks out of the way as, relative to home birth's advantages, they just aren't important. When a woman gives birth in safe, supportive familiar surroundings, birth is very different to the way it's presented on *One Born Every Minute*, where the women giving birth often feel helpless and panicky. She'll vocalise for sure, but the sounds are low and deep, in due course grunty and guttural. Even from a neighbouring room, you wouldn't hear much. And besides, you're engaged in the most magnificent act of your life, so I assure you that what the neighbours think will be the last thing on your mind. As for mess, this is a myth. A few wet towels, a bit of blood. Birth at home leaves behind nothing you couldn't sort with a bin bag and a hot wash, so put it out of your mind.

---

their baby early in pregnancy. Others may start thinking about it at 36 weeks. At whatever point in pregnancy you become interested, begin with a chat with a community or home birth team midwife. You're bound to have lots of questions, as will your partner, and you'll likely want these answering before taking your plan forward.

If you opt late on to change from care in hospital to care at home, never be deterred by the concern that it would be administratively complicated, or that there would be too much to organise.

Confidence builds over time, so it's entirely normal for women to reach the decision to give birth at home in the last trimester. It will be simple to switch tracks as long as you make contact with the community team swiftly. In most cases, the midwives who'll be supporting you will be nothing short of delighted to welcome you on board.

If your new plan necessitates a switch of hospitals (boundaries sometimes mean a booking hospital doesn't cover your area for home birth), don't be put off by what is, in the scheme of things, a tiny bureaucratic blip – transferring your care across will be fairly seamless once you've made your intentions clear.

There may be a good reason why another hospital doesn't suit you, especially as you will need to factor in the possibility of transfer. But resist parking your home birth plan merely because your current hospital has come to feel familiar. You may well have got used to it, but it remains a public institution where the chance of you meeting a midwife more than once is slight. The reassurance you may feel about a hospital where you've had a handful of antenatal appointments doesn't come close to the safety, comfort and all-round ease you'll feel from being cared for in your own home.

You can usually obtain a number for your hospital's

Mothers with a toddler or older children often dismiss giving birth at home for no other reason than the fear that their little ones would be distressed by the experience. But the body is wise, and usually saves up labouring for the wee hours when its work won't be disturbed. The likeliest eventuality is that children sleep right though, waking to find they've a surprise with their breakfast. Even if they are awake, or the birth takes place in the daytime, children rarely seem bothered by the sounds or their mum's behaviour, to the point where it's almost as if they recognise it. If you consider that children would have witnessed birth for thousands of years, it's perhaps not too far-fetched to imagine that calm acceptance might be a natural, inbuilt response to an event that is, after all, very normal – and that our modern-day anxiety is actually the stranger expectation of the two. That said, a child waking up and a child being present are two different things, and if you think you'd feel distracted or disturbed by your child or children being around, simply make sure you have a robust childcare plan.

community team by going to their website, where there may be an online option to self-refer. Alternatively, call the hospital switchboard for the community team office number, or, if you've plenty of time, ask your midwife at your next appointment. The community midwife may then visit you at home, and go through everything with you. If you get in touch and don't hear back within 48 hours, always make a follow-up call to make sure your message has been received and the wheels are in motion.

Provision

Home birth services vary around the country. Theoretically, every woman is entitled to choose and receive midwife support to birth at home but, in practice, some areas have a more reliable, easy-to-access service than others. Cycles – both vicious and virtuous – predictably establish themselves, with women being discouraged and not following up where service seems sketchy, while strong, well-supported community midwife teams and mothers hearing from other mothers how wonderful it is, result in demand and supply thriving.

Lack of support can range from mothers being pushed from pillar to post regarding booking-in, to eleventh-hour obstacles being placed in the way, such as being told that there are staff shortages and that a midwife in labour can't be guaranteed.

On a forward-looking note, things are changing. The recent national maternity review, Better Births, acknowledged the need for greater levels of personalised care and continuity of care in the maternity service, and work is underway to make this a reality.

Caseload midwifery is one proposed plan, and would be an efficient and effective way to meet both goals. One midwife is designated her own caseload of women, supporting them from first appointment, through pregnancy, to birth. Development of dedicated home birth teams is another route – mothers and midwives get to know each other over time, and to form familiar, trusting relationships, which are the long-acknowledged bedrock of a positive birth experience.

Certain areas already have these systems in place, along with some fairly eye-opening statistics to confirm that they work. Sussex (9% home birth rate compared to 2.1% nationally), Powys, Wales (8%), Dorset (6%) and also Windsor, South Devon, Sussex, and Southwark in London all offer very high standards of community care to local mothers, and take active steps to promote home birth as a safe and viable option for women at low risk of complications. Previous theories that linked low home birth rates to socio-economic status of an area, or even age of mothers, now need to be set aside in the light of new evidence.

High rates of home birth show up when home birth has been offered as a realistic option, so NHS CCGs (Clinical Commissioning Groups) exploring how to take the National Maternity Review recommendations forward should look at these glowing examples of gold standard care and learn from their methods and models.

So be hopeful. And should you encounter problems when trying to book for a home birth, don't be discouraged. If expectations rise, better standards will follow. Take the stance of a consumer, examine the ts and cs and require and request that your service provider duly provides.

A friend of mine was told at one of her last midwife appointments that there was a chance a midwife wouldn't be available when she went into labour as some of the team were on holiday. And so it proved – they called up when she was in labour and were told they'd have to go into hospital. She was completely thrown by it, and ended up having a really terrible experience. I decided to learn from it, and to forestall any such nonsense by addressing it directly in an early appointment. I didn't want to scupper the trust that had been building, but I wanted my midwives to be fully aware that my home birth plan wasn't for sale – that I wasn't prepared to be subject to last-minute variables, save genuinely medical ones; I made it clear that I saw it as their responsibility to attend me and that I would be expecting them to attend me in labour. I made sure the conversation was recorded in my notes too. I brought it up twice more, just to be very clear of my position and I followed it up with a letter to the head of midwifery at my local hospital.

It's a shame the service's reliability was even in question, but as it was, they were entirely there for me when I needed them, and were brilliant. I think until there's enough demand, those of us who are really clear on home birth as a choice need to pave the way and put the legal and ethical onus squarely on the service to support us.

Jane

The midwives' regulator, the Nursing and Midwifery Council (NMC), makes it clear that midwives should support women's informed choice, even if that means the midwife has to improve her training or skills or if her employer claims that it does not have the resources. It states that the denial of a home birth service affects women just as much as denying them a hospital birth would (NMC Circular 8-2006).

Though there is now no legal obligation for a local health authority to provide a midwife to attend a home birth, you still have the right to birth at home, and there are no laws forcing you to go to hospital. If you find your health authority unsupportive, persevere. Write a letter to the head of midwifery, explaining that it is your intention to give birth at home and that you require a midwife to attend you, reminding them that it is government policy that the NHS should support a woman who intends to give birth at home, where clinically appropriate.

Copy in the chief executive, even your local MP if you feel

like it and, if necessary, enlist the support of AIMS (Association for the Improvement of Maternity Services) and Birthrights. org. Both organisations offer free advice and are experienced and knowledgeable about your rights and health authority responsibilities. Attend local home birth and Positive Birth groups as well, as mother-to-mother support will help you to feel confident about your request and encouraged to get the care you need in place. In reality, it's rare that you will need to negotiate at a high level to get what you need, but if you do find yourself bang in the middle of a home birth black hole, doggedly pursue your home birth wish and don't give up. According to AIMS and the support site homebirth. org, when women stick to their guns, midwife care at home is usually arranged.

Independent care

An alternative route to NHS midwifery care is to book an independent midwife. Not private midwifery services from a private birth centre: a fully qualified, entirely independent midwife, registered with IMUK, who has chosen to work outside the NHS in a self-employed capacity.

Midwives working in this way (they often work in partnerships or groups) have greater freedom to practise individualised, woman-focused care as compared to NHS midwifery, which is more restricted by guidelines and protocols. They will also be in a position to guarantee continuity of care, the benefits of which are well documented. They give care to a woman and her family through pregnancy and the same midwife cares for the woman as she births her baby and supports the family afterwards.

Independent midwives are still regulated by the NMC and are required to regularly update their training and practice. It may seem like a large outlay, but it would be a shame to rule this route out before weighing the care with the cost. Fees range from £3,000 to £5,000, which covers care in pregnancy, being on call, attending you in labour and postnatal support until your baby is a month old. Most independent midwives reduce their fees in cases of low income and also offer instalment plans. Go to imuk.org.uk to find independent midwives in your area and research the new caseload schemes, like Neighbourhood Midwives.

Your choice

If you have complex issues in pregnancy and are under consultant care because you have been classed as high risk, you still have a right to a home birth if this is your informed choice. You are responsible for making decisions about where you give birth, and if, after exploring the risks and benefits of giving birth in hospital as well as home, home feels preferable, you are entitled to midwife support like anyone else.

The risks of each situation will vary; further, the perception of risk is personal. So whether you have a high BMI, a previous caesarean, a breech baby, or a history of a particular health issue, you'll need to see up-to-date evidence, request written details of your local guidelines, read up on research and factor in your own personal experience and feelings in order to weigh up the pros and cons of each setting.

Don't allow routine policies to dictate your choices, as there are other factors to consider. For example, a labour ward setting is recommended for women with a history of caesarean, due to the risk of scar rupture (0.15%). But labour at home can often be quick and efficient, meaning the scar is less taxed. As well as that, you would have the undivided, undistracted attention of one skilled midwife, which provides a very high level of safety. So make sure to use the meetings, current evidence-based information, as well as your own

Home birth: a human right

Under the Human Rights Act 1998, all UK public bodies must respect the rights set out in the European Convention on Human Rights. Public bodies include all NHS institutions. This means that NHS bodies must respect human rights when making decisions. It also means that caregivers working for public bodies must respect human rights as they go about their work.

Article 8 of the European Convention on Human Rights protects every person's right to respect for their autonomous choice about their private life. In Ternovszky v Hungary (2010), the European Court found that this includes women's right to decide the circumstances, and location, in which they give birth. Article 8 is a qualified right. Respect for private life and autonomous choices can be limited only if there are genuinely legitimate reasons for doing so and these are proportionate.

But the public body refusing to respect a person's choice would have to prove both the reasons for limiting choice and that these are proportionate. If an NHS Trust refuses to provide a home birth service, this may breach your Article 8 rights unless it can give good reasons for its decision, which must be backed up by evidence. Further to this, the legal principle of consent means that you cannot be compelled to give birth in any particular location or medical setting against your will, so long as you have mental capacity to make your own decisions. If staffing shortages are given as a reason for refusing your choice of place of birth, a hospital may be expected to have contingency plans in place (such as hiring independent midwives) to ensure that there are enough staff to provide the services it has promised.

If you have been told by your midwife or other healthcare professionals during your pregnancy that you can give birth at home, you may have a 'legitimate expectation' of giving birth there. This is simply a legal way of saying that you should get what you have been promised. It is only lawful to refuse to honour a legitimate expectation if there are proportionate reasons for doing so.

Midwives have a 'duty of care' to attend women at home. Any midwife who withdraws care from a woman will be held professionally accountable for their decision. This means the midwife could face disciplinary sanctions by the NMC for failing to attend a home birth. Local Supervising Authority midwifery officers, supervisors of midwives and midwifery managers have a professional duty to support midwives to provide home births.

If you are advised against giving birth at home because you are high risk, you cannot be compelled to attend hospital. Midwives are under a professional obligation to respect a woman's decision to give birth outside hospital. You are responsible for making your decisions about where you give birth. Your decision cannot lawfully be overridden by anyone else unless you lack mental capacity to make decisions about your healthcare.

Your midwife and hospital consultant, if you have one, should work with you to put in place a care plan that makes it possible for you to exercise your choice to give birth at home. Healthcare professionals must present information about birth choices in an unbiased and objective way. If a woman has made a decision in response to coercion or threats, including the threat of involvement of social services, she may not have given her consent to treatment, and the healthcare professional may be legally liable for failing to obtain consent. If a healthcare professional has breached their duty of care, they can be referred to their regulatory body.

pregnancy-honed instincts to weigh the risks and inform your plan.

You should also seek out people who've been in the same situation and hear their experience. Go to tellmeagoodbirthstory.com to find details of women with a whole range of birth experiences.

Once you've gathered your thoughts, meet with the head of midwifery or a midwife manager in your local maternity ward to talk your options through. In such a situation, it would be worth considering hiring a doula, or even looking into a one-to-one consultation with an independent midwife, to get an impartial opinion. With prior discussion and a specialised care plan, healthcare teams can often be sympathetic and supportive, so don't discount yourself from the off.

My first birth was straightforward, but my second ended in a caesarean. For my third I wanted to give birth at home, as my first labour had been very easy, and it seemed the logical route. But when I went to talk to the supervisor of midwifery about it, she talked me through what she said would be a safer, more sensible plan. It all sounded great at the time.

They said if there was a need to transfer from home, because of an issue with the scar, it would be hugely disruptive and distressing for me (I didn't know at the time how incredibly unlikely scar rupture was), and what would I think if they were able to provide me with a quiet, comfortable room in the birth centre, along with a birth pool.

It all sounded like a great compromise in the moment. But oh my God, what a mad, misguided plan it turned out to be. For starters, it completely overlooked the very great likelihood that as a third-time mother with a previously swift birth, I was probably going to give birth quickly again, so the chances of me using that nice calm birth pool were tiny. Secondly, I later learned that the risk of scar rupture was highest during dilation – and that was when attentive midwife care was imperative.

As it was, my waters broke, contractions were powerful from the off, and the hour that I laboured I was completely alone save for my husband. He bundled me in the car half-dressed as I was feeling the urge to push, and I ended up falling to my knees in the hospital foyer and giving birth there. How I wish I'd listened to my instincts – or just done more research. I could still have had a hospital plan as back-up, but surely more important than anything would have been having a midwife to call when I needed her. I'm sure their intentions were good, but given they know how women labour, and that subsequent births are often quick, how can a plan like that have been about my safety? Looking back now, I'm sure it was about not wanting to have to explain to those on high why a woman with a previous caesarean was having a home birth.

Amy

Once you book community support, all your antenatal care will take place at home or in your community. You can attend your 12 and 20-week scans as usual, and at your other appointments a midwife offers exactly the same checks as you'd receive in hospital – blood pressure, urine tests and a check on your baby's heart rate. Where community appointments do differ is that they often involve more than just routine observations. There's often a chance to chat and ask questions – about pregnancy, labour, or simply how your day has been.

Some teams are small, comprising four or five midwives, others are larger with 10 or more. Over the course of your pregnancy, it's likely you'll meet most of the midwives on the team, and certainly come to feel as though you have a relationship with the team caring for you overall.

When does your midwife come on the day?

As recently as 60 years ago, we would have had womenfolk around – aunts, sisters, neighbours, grandmothers – a chain of support that meant that right from girlhood, we had a sense of what to expect. We'd have heard birth, maybe seen birth. Above all, vital wisdom about pregnancy and labour would have percolated through without us even thinking about it. When labour began, women around us with experience were on hand to show the way – tacitly decoding the early stages of cramping, or first contractions for example, with a gesture as simple as putting the kettle on.

These days it's different. There's little in the way of a supportive or birth-confident female community and our understanding of what to expect is usually built on other people's scary stories, unsettling television programmes and a smattering of antenatal classes.

There isn't much to draw on in the way of positive first-hand experience, and when things do begin, the lonely reality of your hospital's requirement that you aren't admitted until you're in active labour starts to be felt.

We have come to accept this arrangement as normal. A mother in the early stages of labour is expected to manage alone at home, with a partner who's likely to be feeling equally unsure, and won't be admitted into a birth centre or maternity ward until labour is strong and established.

Guidance on this is scant and mostly unreliable, amounting to over-basic, unhelpful benchmarks like, 'when you are having three contractions in 10 minutes'. As this could easily be happening well in advance of established labour – and as early surges can be very powerful, it's easy for a woman to feel anxious and overwhelmed and to go into hospital 'too' early.

If you've arranged midwife care at home, all this wondering, watching and waiting is avoided. The support you'll have received in pregnancy will have already removed a lot of uncertainty and helped you to feel confident, and now there's the option to feel more of the same. Whether you choose to stay at home or go to hospital to give birth is up to you. The point is that now, when you most need it, there is a knowledgeable midwife to call, who can drop by, check all is well and reassure you that everything is as it should be.

As doula Michelle Gerlis explains:

> Women don't realise how long the build-up to labour can be. It can be a day or even two for first-time mothers – and that's almost certainly going to mean managing a night of cramps or contractions. When women know what to expect, and feel supported with that, they do so with confidence and calm. That's less easy when there's no one to call but a stranger on a hospital triage ward.
>
> When women plan to have a baby at home, they've got their midwife to call, and maybe a doula too. This support – which will give them a sense of where they are, the reassurance that all is normal, as well as all manner of ways to comfort themselves, helps them to manage their expectations, and pace themselves. It's the emotional equivalent of releasing a handbrake and just that bit of support can help her relax.

Having the assurance that a midwife is on hand for the build-up stages of birth can be helpful. And just knowing that support is available often reduces and even erases lingering anxieties anyway. In fact women are often surprised by how confident they feel when the plan is to stay put. They draw huge confidence from being in control of their environment, which in turn helps them feel in control of the birth process.

Being undistracted by questions like when to go to hospital, or the general emotional static that's involved with an unknown set-up or engaging with unfamiliar third parties, makes it possible to concentrate – to focus properly on the normal sensations of birth. The result is that some women don't want a midwife until they're in well-established labour. You might want to put in an advance call informing your midwives that you think things are starting, but, free from the need to think and plan, you will probably be able to attune and feel for yourself the point when you need one to come.

Looking after you in labour

Once you are in established labour, your midwife stays with you. On arrival, she will set up her equipment, usually on a towel or tray in an unobtrusive corner. Scissors and clip for cutting and clamping the cord; absorbent pads for protecting bedding and carpets; back-up breathing equipment for the baby; drugs to stop bleeding; her sonicaid or pinard and, if requested, a bottle of entonox (gas and air).

She needs to get comfortable, to take her shoes off and settle in, so have a place ready where she can sit, rest, and also write notes. Have tea, drinks and snacks to hand – and have your partner prepped to remind her to make herself at home.

From that point, your midwife will take *your* lead. She will need to keep an eye on you and check that things are unfolding normally. And this she will do both with intermittent observations like temperature, pulse and foetal heart rate – but also with her eyes and ears, being with you for periods, and giving you privacy when desired.

Though established labour is usually more predictable time-wise than early labour, it can still take some hours for the body to open and the baby to move down and through and, unless there is no or very little sign of progress, you shouldn't feel rushed or as though you're supposed to have reached a certain point at any time.

So long as you and your baby are well, the care remains constant and those offering it work at the pace of your body. Your midwife is like a trusted travel companion, in the background when you want her to be, alongside when you need her and you just feel and follow each sensation as it strengthens, circles, plateaus and deepens, until finally, the arrival of your baby draws near.

Birth preferences

At home, the care adapts itself around you and your choices. Though your preferences should be paramount wherever you choose to have your baby, the current of hospital care is strong. First wishes easily get washed away by institutional flow, and end up coming second when they push against protocols and a mother feeling the need to cooperate.

Take vaginal examinations. These are used routinely in hospital, to plot progress and in particular as part of the admissions procedure. According to NICE guidelines, they should be offered when a decision needs making. In recent years, it's become a hospital habit to routinely do a vaginal examination in order to 'decide' whether the woman can go to the birth centre or labour ward, a procedure she is entitled to decline.

Some women feel internal examinations to be unnecessary and invasive. Being told you are 4cm dilated is inviting you to self-assess, to consider how 'well' you are doing, and conscious thinking even of this sort can put a brake on hormonal flow and all the vital letting go the mind has to do for labour to unfold with ease.

It may be for this physiological reason that women decline – or there may be more personal reasons. In your own home, you will have developed a trusting relationship with your midwives through pregnancy, meaning your informed decisions will be heard and respected – and vice versa. If a change of plan is necessary, you should feel confident and trust their guidance.

Your personal choices might involve not having vaginal exams, when and how you want to be monitored, or whether or not you want vitamin K for your baby. You may want your midwife to hold your hand or have an express preference for privacy.

Home support helps with advance decisions too, like how long you feel comfortable being pregnant. Recommendations to induce are sometimes heavy-handed. The groundedness and agency you'll feel as a result of being cared for at home will help you to be objective, free of pressure and able to make an informed choice based on what feels right for you.

Your baby arrives

When labour reaches its final stages, a second midwife is called. This is so that there are two pairs of hands available when the baby arrives, and as the midwives will likely know each other, the extra support can be reassuring for everyone. That said, you may like feeling unobserved, or just feel very safe and undisturbed with the midwife who has been caring for you, so it is always your choice as to whether you want the second midwife in the room before your baby starts to arrive.

There is no need to plan a specific spot or room in which to give birth to your baby – that freedom, to see what happens, to go where you feel, to respond spontaneously – is one of the biggest benefits of birthing at home.

You may have a birth pool set up, with a plan to deliver in the water. Or a soft, towel-layered 'nest' set up in your bedroom. But a woman in labour goes where she wants to – and babies come where they come, so having a fixed plan can be a distraction. What does need preparing is a few towels and some instant warmth, either by turning the central heating up, or switching on an electric fan heater.

At home, babies aren't 'delivered'. A midwife will only control and guide your baby's emergence if she sees help is needed or wanted. Otherwise, the care is usually hands-off (as per Royal College of Midwives guidelines), allowing the natural force of contractions and the muscles of your pelvic floor to help the baby advance and wriggle free of your body.

The majority of newly born babies will take their first breath without help. It may take a few seconds, or even a minute or two for the baby's system to fire up, and your midwife will be keeping a close eye, stimulating the baby gently with a rub of a warm towel if she has caught them or, if you are in a pool, covering you both with a towel and doing the same.

You may be in a position, for example on the floor or bed, where you just want to stop and stare at your baby and not necessarily pick them up immediately – and a pause like this is normal, a chance for you to take your baby in. Once your baby starts to breathe and pink up, they may cry for a short burst, and this helps them to stimulate their lungs and clear any remaining fluid.

Delayed cord clamping is now normal practice, and by leaving the cord to pulsate, richly oxygenated blood from the placenta continues to flow into the baby, providing a natural back-up in those first moments. If the baby needs a bit more help, your midwife will be trained and skilled to manage this, and have a bag and valve mask ready if she thinks it is needed. This works in the exact same way as the high-tech resuscitation equipment in hospital.

As midwife Frances Rivers explains:

> *One of people's biggest fears about having a baby at home is the idea that their baby won't breathe. But the chances of a baby needing a significant amount of help to start breathing after a normal labour are very small.* * *Assessment in pregnancy will have already told us that the baby is healthy and physiologically equipped. Checks during labour will have given us assurances on how the baby is coping, right until the end, when we are monitoring very regularly. If we had any cause for concern, the mother would have already been transferred to hospital. If we do need to step in, it's not the same aid you'd give to a grown adult who's heart and lungs had given out. A healthy baby's lungs are brand-new and capable of breathing alone – there's just a bit of shift in pressure they have to manage, and sometimes a bit of stimulation can help with that.*

In due course, your midwife will get you into a comfortable position, adjusting the cord that's still connecting your baby's body to your body, helping you as you take your baby on to your chest, and wrapping you both up warm with towels or a blanket.

During those wonderful first moments, when you and your partner get to take your baby in, your midwife will keep a quiet eye, checking that all is well and that there is no

---

* About 2 in 1000 babies need stimulating to take their first breath in a normal labour and of that 0.2%, around 90% are successfully brought to breathe using a simple bag and mask.

excessive bleeding.

A haemorrhage is more common in a long birth where the uterus has been working for a very long time, or in medicated births, for example where the hormone syntocinon has been used to augment the labour. It is much rarer in natural births where labour has been physiological. Even so, safety measures are in place and the midwife will have an injection of syntometrine or syntocinon drawn up to stop undue bleeding, just in case.

In a natural birth at home, it is usual to wait for the placenta to deliver naturally, though your midwife will have a syntometrine injection ready in case you want the third stage of labour managed. The injection can induce a feeling of wooziness and nausea so, unless there is medical necessity, it is probably worth letting nature take its course. The quiet calm of your home is the perfect setting to allow this, facilitating the last surges of oxytocin that help to deliver the placenta.

The final thing the midwife will do, before getting you comfortable in bed, is a check to see if you need stitches. You can keep your baby in your arms as she does this, but she will need you to lie on your back and will require a good light. If you do need suturing, in most cases your midwife will be able to do it and will administer a local anaesthetic beforehand. Some women find this harder than the birth, so be prepared. It's natural to be a bit tense, but deep inhales of lavender and gas and air, as well as closing your eyes to concentrate or maybe holding a birth partner's hand, will all help and it'll be over in no time.

Finally, it's time to get comfortable. Someone will help you have a quick wash or shower, get into a clean T-shirt or nightdress and some knickers with a sanitary towel – and then you just climb into your readied bed and sink back on the pillow.

There's nothing more to think about. Your partner is

snuggled one side, you've tea and toast on the other, and your baby is cuddled close on your front. As moments go, there is nothing like it in the world!

> *I am passionate about birth at home. At home – safe in their own environment, women are powerful, strong and amazing! Sometimes women or their families worry that 'something will happen' but I reassure them that I'm not a cheerleader. I am a skilled midwife practised in emergency skills with all the necessary equipment. My job is to support, to reassure, to subtly monitor wellbeing of mother and baby and, of course, to act if there is any problem. It is vital that women have support from midwives who understand and trust physiological home birth, who truly respect what each women wants without imposing arbitrary time limits or restrictions.*
>
> *Claire Chaubert, midwife*

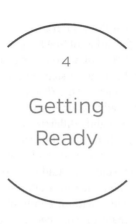

4

Getting Ready

There's a line pregnant women hear all the time. In books, from classes, even from midwives. 'Every birth is different.' It's offered as reassurance, a roundabout way of getting them to manage their expectations and keep an open mind. But it's my feeling that women feel a bit helpless faced with this news, as getting ready for something you've been told is unpredictable can feel sort of pointless.

But the message that birth is a lottery – the signal to keep hope in check and avoid making a plan – isn't just discouraging. It's also untrue. Birth experiences differ. Of course they do. And a flexible mindset has its place. But when women have a suitable setting, labour tends to unfold with relative consistency.

Ironically, for a routine maternity care setting, the warning that birth is a lottery might be more warranted. Though current consensus still considers hospital to be the safest place to have a baby, the multiple variables that are an inherent part of a medical setting – everything from over-lit rooms to shift changes and restrictive protocols – can disturb labour's normal physiological flow. So even with a planned hospital birth, the last thing you'd want to do in preparation is nothing. To have the best chance of a positive experience in hospital, women need to take mindful steps to prepare and be active participants in their birth rather than passive patients.

But what about readying for a birth at home? In your own space, the process is slightly different, as everything you need is already in place. What helps labour to unfold predictably is naturally on hand: privacy, peace and quiet, freedom to move about, control over your surroundings. And a midwife that comes to you, wrapping the care around your body and baby.

Your home provides natural continuity. There are fewer scenarios to anticipate or contingencies to wonder about. Though transfer into hospital certainly needs a think-through, the protective measures and self-management needed for labouring in a place you don't know are now unnecessary. Preparing for birth at home is less about making an action plan, more about working towards a feeling. Over time, and at your own pace, you want to bring your head, heart and body towards an overall sense of 'santosha' – the Sanskrit word for feeling completely comfortable and content. Don't strive for it. It needn't involve effort. Set things up steadily and over a period of time (avoid saving it all up until you finish work, for example) and you'll begin to feel an ease – a calmness of mind and a confident connection with your body. Below are some ideas on how to do that: practical, physical and emotional ways to prepare. And of course, if you do end up in hospital, these tips will have helped prepare you for that too.

Readying for my second birth, at home, was very different to my first birth, which was in hospital. There was a lot of mental and practical preparation first time. I had to kind of gird myself because there was no knowing what to expect. It wasn't the dramatic unexpected so much. It was the strange unfamiliarity of it all – what a hospital feels like at three in the morning, when there's a distant radio playing, a lone cleaner mopping a floor, strangers at a desk chatting casually – the surreal normality of it while you're in the middle of these hugely intense and powerful feelings. It's so jarring and incongruent, and to help it not feel like that, you've got to get yourself solid and ready. Second time, I didn't have any of that to worry about. I didn't have to think about a single thing. When I wanted to take my clothes off I did. When I wanted to hum and moan, it wasn't even a question of 'letting myself' – it just was. There was no staging, no needing to buffer myself from what was going on around me. It was just home.

Mirie

Ditching the headline

Something to consider, if your plan is to birth at home, is to avoid telling anyone you're planning a home birth. Remember our discussion about how loaded the term can be. Even if you aren't met with eye-rolling, announcing you are having a home birth can trigger unhelpful comments like being told you are 'brave', or that you're putting your baby in danger. Our society isn't up to date on the safety of home birth, and it can sap your energy to repeatedly defend your plans. One alternative, if someone asks you where you're having your baby, is to say the name of your booking hospital, or to say 'I'll have a midwife coming to my home and I'm going to see'. This is the truth, after all.

Walk

Walking every day in the last month of pregnancy is valuable in two ways. Firstly it gets your baby into a good position. Physics alone will help the heaviest part of the baby – its head – to shift south. But adding some gravity will counterbalance all the seated hours we spend and help the baby to drop deeper still. Having your baby well down in the pelvis means that when the time comes, his or her crown is more likely to be pressing heavily onto the cervix, helping labour to start spontaneously and unfold normally. Secondly, the ritual of a daily walk readies you mentally. The simple ceremony of walking 20 minutes away from your house, and 20 minutes back, works multiple miracles – bringing your breath into rhythm with your body, clearing your crowded head of busy thoughts and planting you in the present, just as you will be in birth.

Pregnancy yoga

This is another weekly ritual to benefit from. It's not about getting fit, though flexibility and strength will be a bonus. It's about learning how to lengthen and widen; relaxing to order; becoming familiar with a different, more instinctive side to yourself. You'll learn to breathe and make shapes with your body as you instinctively will in labour, so getting accustomed in advance can be a fantastic help. Patterns of tension hold our bodies in place. But in yoga you get to unravel those, to find space and give, resilience and release – all at the same time.

Yoga is a weekly reminder that birth is a matter of letting your baby out, not getting your baby out. Classes that have a birth preparation component, led by a teacher with first-hand experience of birth, will be the most useful, for example, Active Birth, Yogabirth, Birthlight or Daisy Birthing. There is often tea and talk at the end, and this chance to share and talk as a circle of women can also help you to feel confident.

Imagine it

It's probably best not to have too fixed an idea about exactly where to give birth at home. But it can be helpful visualising it generally – picturing yourself labouring in your kitchen for example, or lying in the bath. For one it's intention-strengthening. Creating a clear mental picture can help it become concrete. But it's also good for considering the 'nest' or 'position' potential of various spaces in your home.

Where would you be comfortable? Where could you feel private or enjoy some company? You'll want the chance to focus and it's good to imagine where – hanging from your headboard; standing in your shower; sitting back to front on the toilet; retreating to the dark, cosy spare room at the back of the house. It might make sense to your conscious, non-labouring mind to install the birth pool in your sunlit conservatory. But the female mammal in you is likely to prefer the tiny downstairs loo. So keep in mind that labour is an involuntary process and helped when it has the chance to be just that.

Have lots of pillows at the ready, perhaps candles and fairylights for instant mood, and then see what feels good on the day. You can ground your mental pictures by writing positive affirmations on pieces of paper and sticking them up around the house. Try 'Each wave is bringing me closer to my baby', or 'My body knows what to do'. Absorbing these messages beforehand can provide a guide rope for when you're in labour later. Rooting and reassuring, they become unconscious instructions that your body will naturally follow.

Raspberry leaf tea and other goodness

Drinking a cup of raspberry leaf tea every day from 29 weeks can help prepare the body for birth. 'Raspberry leaf is a very gentle herb but it can be powerful when it's had a chance to build up in the body,' says medical herbalist Jo Dunbar, of traditional herbal apothecary, Botanica Medica. 'Regular consumption of raspberry leaf tea in the final months of pregnancy can aid delivery because it helps to tone the muscles of the uterus, meaning they are primed and ready to contract.' If possible, buy the loose herb as it is more potent than the bagged alternative. Regularly eating dates from 37 weeks has proven benefits for labour and taking vitamin C and garlic capsules throughout pregnancy will help to prevent Group B strep and urine infections.'

Gather good stories

Birth confidence is built on good stories, so go gathering them. Talk to women who've had positive experiences having their babies and see how it makes you feel: you will probably feel reassured. And excited. Probably curious too. Even a single positive exchange can make a huge difference. Ordinary know-how on what to expect and how to help yourself is really enabling.

Attend your nearest free Positive Birth group (positivebirth.org), or request a birth buddy to email from tellmeagoodbirthstory.com – and if you know a friend or a colleague with a positive story to share, take her for a coffee and ply her with questions. Network on social media and fill your heart and head with as much good mother-to-mother wisdom as you can. The message 'I did it, so can you' is a magic key.

Eat well

In pregnancy, eating well can help you to feel well and prepared for the birth. Steer clear of processed food and eat fresh, big-flavoured, nutrient-filled meals you feel confident building a baby from: porridge with blueberries, poached eggs, spring vegetable and barley soup, roast chicken, butternut squash risotto, baked salmon, garlic potatoes, berry and banana smoothies, fresh tomato salsa, mashed avocado on toast, almonds, apples, homemade cake, good-quality chocolate, roasted vegetables, full-fat milk, loads of dates, buttered wholegrain bread and honey. Good food will increase your vitality and energy, and there are big emotional benefits too – home cooking is a wonderful way to ready your nest before birth.

Relaxation

When I asked the mothers of tellmeagoodbirthstory.com what helped them most to prepare for home birth, they said relaxation. In the weeks beforehand, many of them regularly set aside some special time to relax: lowering the lights and lying on their bed to slow and settle their breath, or listening to a hypnobirthing recording, or lighting some candles and having a warm bath.

As well as being a lovely way to nourish you in pregnancy, a relaxation ritual sets up a super signal – habituating your muscles to a voice, or a mood, or a set of messages so that when you need to unwind on demand, you can and will.

Get familiar with what it feels like to unknit your brow, to soften the muscles around your eyes, to empty out your shoulders. Visualise balloons attached to your hands – and imagine them floating up and away. Hypnobirthing is now a tried and tested tool for relaxing in birth, so attend a local course or invest in a DVD or download. Or create your own little relaxation ritual, by playing birdsong, or softly lapping waves on your earphones (available on many free white noise apps), lying on your back or side in a warm, quiet, prepared space, closing your eyes, and relaxing each part of your body in turn.

In the last weeks of pregnancy I loved using this visualisation. As I breathed in, I imagined taking up any discomfort, stress, negativity and pain with it – letting it disperse up and above me, into the sky, right up into the blue that's above the clouds... and then as I breathed down, clean, clear warm light washed through my body bringing my baby with it. In labour, it was no effort to imagine and felt like the most natural thing in the world. It helped me hugely, and allowed me to meet each contraction with great calm.

Eilidh

Birth wishes

Over the course of your pregnancy, you'll have got clear on the biology of birth – what helps labour to happen. And you'll already be aware of how you work as a person, and what is likely to soothe and support you in labour. Meeting these needs will help you feel safe and allow baby-bringing oxytocin to flow – so write them down in a wish-list. This is all a birth plan is really, a contract of preferences which strengthens intention, and informs carers what's important to you. It can list whether or not you want vaginal examinations; if and how often your baby's heart rate will be monitored; if you want a natural or a managed third stage; the way you want to welcome your baby; if you want your baby to have vitamin K and in what way.

I often suggest that women write it like a letter – a friendly welcome and thank you to start, followed by a simple wish list – and then put one copy on your fridge for easy reading, and one in your notes.

It will be useful to think a bit about after the birth too, ways to plan and protect the precious first fortnight when you'll be needing to rest and focus on feeding and getting to know your baby. To avert a flurry of texts and requests to visit right after your baby's arrival, inform friends and family in advance that you'll get in touch with them when you're ready.

If it's your second or subsequent child, make sure you have thought through what to do with your child or children. You may be quite happy for them to be around on the day, leaving them to sleep if it's nighttime or joining in if they want to. But if you feel their presence will distract you, get a good childcare plan in place by enlisting a neighbour or nearby friend for instant help, or family if there's more time.

As you travel through pregnancy, reading, listening to stories, and getting a feel for what you need, consider carefully what kind of support you want for your birth at home. Some people may feel their partner and midwife will be enough. Others may have a large community team, with less opportunity to know their midwife, so someone extra to support you in labour may be a helpful addition.

Besides this, the build-up to labour needs navigating too. It can often be a day or two for first-time mothers, and if you and your partner are alone during this time, or at least without emotional and practical guidance on how to pace yourself, it can feel a bit lonely. A doula or friend or family member who knows about birth can provide valuable reassurance in the early stages, distracting you, reminding you all is normal and, if there's a night to get through, settling you in bed with a hot water bottle. An extra pair of hands can be useful later too, for filling a birth pool, rubbing your back, or making tea. Look online for a doula in your area (doula.org.uk) or ask at your local home birth or Positive Birth group.

Stuff

You don't need much to have a baby at home. A stack of towels is essential and easily obtained by asking friends and family to donate the oldest in their possession. A couple of old sheets and a cheap shower curtain can be useful too, to create pathways, have under the birth pool and prevent things getting wet – and these need stacking in a corner, easily to hand.

Plastic or polythene sheeting is often recommended, but it's not the cosiest feel and the sound of sticking feet on it might end up driving you mad. One reason labouring at home feels good is because it's your space – so beware of too much stuff that might make it feel like a 'facility'. This includes the birth pool. For first births, consider waiting until labour is well-established and underway before inflating it (unless it's well out of the way), as it can compromise your patience having it staring at you for days in advance.

I bounced on my ball in the kitchen for the first part of my birth, but when the time came to concentrate, I went directly to my bedroom and got the most wonderful surprise. My lovely hub had created this amazing soft floor arrangement, using lots of cushions, throws, sheets and an old duvet. It was fairylit too and looked like a bedouin tent. The feeling of being able to just throw myself down and get comfortable was amazing.

Marie

It's a good idea to build a coping kit – a little treasure trove of comforts installed by your bedside – and details on this are in the next chapter. You'll also need lots of pillows; a cosy blanket or two; a yoga mat for knee support; a birth ball for bouncing on or an ironing board with a pillow for leaning on; absorbent bed-pads; kitchen towel and bin liners; a bucket (it's normal to be sick once or twice in labour), bendy straws for drinking, candles or fairylights; an electric heater (for instant warmth once the baby is born); an electric fan if it's summer; a torch for the midwife to see in the pool, and if possible an anglepoise lamp in case suturing is required afterwards. Also, consider creating a makeshift sling by suspending a knotted sheet from a banister, or throwing it over the top of a door and shutting it firm. It can feel great hanging off something firm and letting your lower half go.

If you have big, brightly-lit spaces, you might want to consider ways to black out the windows, either by nailing up a dark sheet or covering them with black paper or newspaper. And for your own comfort, have loose clothes to wear (big T-shirts, a towelling dressing gown), warm socks, a few pairs of large knickers, some big maternity pads, clothes and nappies for the baby, and a hospital bag packed just in case.

Refreshment-wise, freeze whole grapes and also some fruit juice in an icecube tray (e.g. watermelon, orange). In the moment, something cold and delicious can be spirit-lifting. Have tea, snacks and biscuits for those supporting you and, most important of all, something celebratory for afterwards – a big homemade BIRTH-day cake, or a bottle of champagne.

Birth pools

Warm water in labour is a wonderful thing. The relief of sinking down into a birth pool can feel extraordinary. Installing a pool in your home is not complicated, so never let it be an obstacle when deciding whether or not to give birth at home. Just be aware that less is more, and that a smaller pool is easy to erect, quick to fill, and no trouble to empty and clear away.

There are plenty of birth pool companies now, but also find out if your local home birth group or hospital loan them out. If this is the case, you only have to pay for a liner.

Make sure you have everything you need for inflating it,

filling it, and draining it: electric pump and drainer, hose, tap adapters and bucket. And make sure you do a road-test! It's amazing how many leave this to the last minute and discover their designer bath taps don't match the screw-on adapter. You don't want to end up having to bandage everything with gaffa tape.

On a final – slightly contradictory – note, be aware that you don't actually need a birth pool to have a baby at home. Today natural birth seems to have become synonymous with birthing in water, but though it can be a soothing aid, immersing yourself in a pool is not vital for working your way through labour.

> *For me, arranging and installing a birth pool would have been to make my home a little abnormal, unfamiliar even. I didn't want one single thing in my environment to change – that was why I chose to have my baby at home in the first place, for everything to feel normal and mine. I wanted to keep things really, really simple, just to head to my bedroom when things accelerated and turn out the lights. I knew I had my shower, and a bath if needs be – what I didn't want was all the decisions that seem to come with birth pools – when to put it up, the faff of filling it – and that becoming a distraction. My doula told me that when asked if there was ever a reason not to use a birth pool, the obstetrician who founded the whole waterbirth idea, Michel Odent, said, 'Yes – when birth is going well'!*
>
> *Kavita*

Take it easy

In the last weeks of pregnancy, slow down. Work to the pace of your body. Curious feelings can arise during this period

– intense bursts of energy, bouts of tearfulness, heightened contentment. You also may feel uncomfortable or very tired. Whatever is going on, these emotions are inviting you to listen and, if you're not stopping work until a fortnight before your due date, you won't hear them. So do less. Rest more. Venerate your vulnerability and gentle your way through the days by doing simple things, like folding and putting away baby clothes, cleaning out kitchen cupboards, learning lullabies, or cooking and filling your freezer. Nest in the lovely knowledge that here, at home, is where you're going to give birth to your baby and take all the precious time you need to be aware of where you are – on the threshold of becoming a mother.

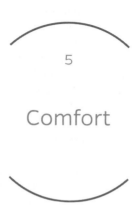

5

Comfort

Having a baby at home provides a beautiful in-built benefit – the chance to frame the sensations of labour, as they are felt by you. Today that's a rare experience. In medical training, doctors are taught that pain is 'what a person says it is'. But from what I've seen, the pain of labour is more often what *other* people say it is.

Current negativity and fear around childbirth makes pain its main argument – the physical 'proof' that birth is something to dread. During pregnancy, it's easy to become convinced of this, thanks to scary birth stories, or TV programmes presenting birth as agony, and the tension and resistance this fear-conditioning creates affects how mothers approach and cope with labour.

But if stories like these are what you've heard, listen carefully to them. When someone has experienced labour as suffering, ask questions. What position were they in? Did they feel safe or exposed? Were they given quiet? In other words, wonder whether it was birth that felt overwhelming, or the conditions in which the mother was trying to manage.

A body in labour *can* feel like a body in combat when the mother is missing what she most needs: a quiet, intimate environment; attuned, compassionate care; and a steady flow of comforts. At home, where this is all readily on tap, it can be a very different story.

When I conducted a survey on tellmeagoodbirthstory. com and asked mothers: 'If you had your first baby at home, would you do it again?', a whopping 98 per cent said they would. Far from depleting, most women find giving birth at home completing, so much so that they want to relive it. They describe labour as intense and powerful, arduous in the manner of extreme physical challenge.

Birth is demanding and it will always exact its share of sweat, effort and even tears. But fright isn't an inevitable response to that. Female mammals don't naturally regard their body or baby as a threat, and neither do *human* female mammals when the birthing instinct can fully articulate itself and the mother is enabled to feel and follow the birth with her whole self.

The act of giving birth to a baby has the potential to be a woman's greatest life experience. It was mine – twice – and I gave birth to both my son and daughter at home. It wasn't a choice. It felt like the only way for me, as the birth stories I'd heard from friends and family in hospital sounded negative and the things that happened to them unnecessary.

To me, a medical environment couldn't be less suitable for an act where you have to trust your body. Glaring lights, strangers, sterile delivery rooms, experts managing your behaviour. Even the traditional position of a woman lying on her backside. How can any woman let go in such circumstances? Birth isn't supposed to be clean, logical, controlled by machines or directed by strangers. A woman needs a dark, intimate space, where she is in her element – surrounded by people she loves and trusts. And that's home.

In your own home, you just feel comfortable. Childbirth is dynamic, the sensations and emotions change moment to moment, and you have to be able to concentrate completely to follow that. You can't be civilised, or polished – it can't be thought through. It works on an entirely different register, involving your deepest, instinctive self. To me even a birth pool felt contrived – like a repository for a woman's biological urges, a way to contain birth and all that comes with it. Why? What for? I squatted on my bedroom floor to deliver both my children – because that's what my body wanted me to do.

Kavita

Breathe, move, sigh, sing

There's no need to learn specific birthing positions in labour, or to practise and prepare special breathing techniques, although all mothers are different and some are drawn to this type of preparation. A home environment tends to bring out the best in a mother's body naturally and labour can be felt for what it is. A need. You rely on your body messaging you when you're tired, or when you're hungry. And birth is no different. If you listen to your body, it will tell you what to do.

At the outset, when you're feeling cramps or crampy-waves, leaning on the kitchen counter may feel good, or taking a walk – you could even do some baking! My mum told me how, in the old days, the midwife would get you to read a book while hanging over the side of the bath. It can take a few hours, a full day and even a further night for the feelings to strengthen, and when they do demand more focus, you'll seek comfort more actively – for example by lying on your side with a hot water bottle, thighs, knees and feet propped apart with pillows. Or taking a long, warm shower. Or hanging off your bed's headboard.

If you feel safe and unscrutinised, your breathing is likely to slow and lengthen naturally and, in time, turn to sighs and low moans. You'll move freely, breathe deeply and mark out soothing rhythms by rocking, swaying, or silently counting.

All this gives your body what it needs: the chance to loosen and unload tension; to open and and create space; a steady supply of oxygen and, as things develop, the deep, dreamlike ease brought on by building endorphins.

When your body is well met, birth becomes a set of simple messages. Rest! Bounce! Breathe out! Swing your hips! When difficult, more demanding or even demoralising moments come, delegate. Allow your body to lift you up and over it and it will usually pass. Each new turning point will immerse you more deeply and the world around you will drop away.

Giving birth at home felt so unhurried. And in terms of coping, that was such a help. My first baby was born in hospital, and somehow all the measurement and plotting of progress made me more aware of what each contraction was costing me. But at home, there was none of that – I just waited to see where the next breath took me. Those breaths became ahhhs and in the end, all I could do was let out these long, loud deep sounds from the deepest point of my belly. It felt great. At home, the stronger it got, the bolder I felt – because it took my body over. I remember feeling this craving for frozen clementine segments – they were like nectar. Then once I was in the pool, I found all I wanted to do was stare at the shiny metal of my kettle – to just stare and stare at it until a contraction passed.

Emily

There's a reassuring simplicity to letting labour lead. Awaiting and being guided by your body's cues brings control. Whereas going to hospital necessitates planning and decision-making, in the safe, predictable environment of your home, there's nothing to do but relax and get comfortable – to wait for the magnificent independence of the body to do its work.

If things unfold in a straightforward fashion – and they likely will – you'll feel a pattern emerging, whether you choose to measure contractions and know how dilated you are, or not. When there are no distractions, labour's rhythm becomes clear and, if you feel safe and supported, you'll breathe, move, sing and sigh in step with it. This is your foundation. Besides that, you might want to consider some of the extra tips and tricks listed below – things that have helped women in labour across cultures and forever. (And of course, if you do go to hospital at any point, all these things can help you in that environment too.)

Your comfort kit

At home, managing the sensations of labour doesn't require an arsenal of coping techniques. It's about responding to each feeling – when it comes, in whatever way it comes. In your own space, labour is what it is – a series of non-threatening physical sensations that are just a normal, necessary by-product of your baby being born.

Comfort is all around you at home. There's your own warm, soft bed. A shower you know the heat and force of. Natural opportunities for distraction while your body is readying. And privacy and quiet when you need to focus and give birth.

Feeling and following the waves where you want, in the way you want, means you're less likely to attach emotion to them. Safe and undisturbed, you're unlikely to be scoring them on intensity, or assessing where you are. You'll just be in it – on it – *with it* – seeing what soothes as each feeling unfolds. Your own surroundings provide natural resources, without the need to do anything extra: your own pillows and duvet; the freedom to walk around naked; your own clean toilet; darkness when desired. But besides this, consider building yourself a little comfort kit. Find a basket or box, a proper container to order things in, as if everything's thrown in a bag it can be hard to find what you need. My suggestions for things to include, from my experience of supporting women in birth, are as follows.

Lavender oil
Lavender oil can be inhaled directly from a handkerchief or scarf. The smell may help you relax and feel calmer, and it is also an active analgesic. Besides this, breathing lavender in labour can provide the three-fold focus US doula Penny Simkin says is the key to coping well. With a lavender-infused comforter, her renowned three Rs – ritual, rhythm and relaxation – are all in place:

1. You repeatedly return to it
2. You're breathing rhythmically as you use it
3. Dropping it is your cue to relax.

Frankincense oil
This is another useful oil to have handy as its earthy, potent smell may put a stop to uneven breathing or panic. Breathe its grounding aroma, again on a square of soft cloth, and you'll feel steadied and restored.

Handkerchiefs and flannels
Make sure to have a couple of large, cotton handkerchiefs in your basket, to carry the oils above. Muslin squares are an alternative, as is a favourite headscarf. Just be sure they're soft. You could tuck a couple of flannels (facecloths) in too, as these can be useful in active labour when you may feel hot. Soaked in ice-cold water, and applied to a warm cheek, they will feel amazing.

Warm socks
Women in labour often have cold feet as labour progresses, so warm socks can feel comforting.

Hot water bottles and heat packs
Hot water bottles or heat packs can be a great comfort, so pop two in your basket, preferably mini children's ones as they are easily held in place. In the early stages, the spread of warmth will allow you to sleep and when contractions become powerful and the birth is really underway, a hot water bottle on your lower back can feel fantastic. Whoever's on refill duty should add a little cold water, so that they're not scalding, and make sure they have a cover. Stick-on heat packs are also useful and are available in most chemists.

Camomile tea
Quality, loose-leaf, yellow-headed camomile, from a herbal supplier, can really instil calm – especially if it's tepid and has a teaspoon of honey stirred in. A warm cup of camomile tea can refresh and ready you for whatever your body's bringing.

Pre-prepared massage oil
Essential oils in labour are therapeutic. Have a birth partner use them as part of a soothing massage, and you'll feel deep

ease. Mix your own elixir, using any of the following in an almond or olive oil carrier: rose, geranium, neroli, clary sage, jasmine, mandarin, grapefruit. The smell will change the atmosphere in the room too, and help those caring for you to relax.

Eyemask and earplugs

In their own home, women sometimes continue to talk and engage while in labour. It doesn't mean they're actively 'alert', just so relaxed and uninhibited that they can switch to autopilot. Others retreat and close off completely. Either way, an eyemask, earplugs, a cotton shawl or earphones streaming a relaxation recording are useful to have to hand and can take things to a whole new safe and disinhibiting level. Nearly everyone is pulled inward eventually, even if it's only for the last 10 minutes, and some women are so sensitive to disturbance that just having a midwife in the room, or hearing the birth pool being filled, can be distracting. So make sure birth partners are aware, and have them provide protection for you to focus if you're feeling in any way observed, self-conscious or irritable.

Soften and soothe the senses

There are many things you can do to soothe yourself in birth. There are sensory tricks, like diving into an elevating scent, or being comforted by someone's touch. And there are psychological tools, for example a visualisation or repeating a hypnobirthing affirmation to yourself. Both can work wonders for holding you firm and keeping you steady.

Your lower body is working hard, but consider what other parts of your body you can relax. Your jaw. Your shoulders. Opening and stretching your hands? A cold flannel on your chest or brow for example, or a nice stretch of your back by hanging off your bannister. Once labour is progressing, you and your caregivers will create a kind of alchemy together – repeating, removing and replacing different comforts as seems fit and feels good for you.

Other ideas to consider beyond your basic kit are: a soft ball to squeeze or a smooth stone to hold (a place to 'put' the contraction); sweets to chew; a handheld fan (a breeze in labour is bliss); a cold water atomiser; a very cold flannel on your brow or cheek; ice to crunch; frozen grapes or frozen fruit ice-cubes; juice or coconut water with a straw; a tennis ball (have someone roll it up and down your spine).

Every one of these serves the same aim – a place to put your focus. Partners can get creative, layering comfort upon comfort to cocoon you or, if you hit a dip, bringing in something new to change the energy and boost spirits.

A warm bath can bring profound relief at any point in birth. In order to get really comfortable, consider running it low so that you can fully lie down on your side and keep warm by running a shower head from your shoulders to your feet and back again. Kneeling on all fours is another good bath position. Or you can just fill the bath full, rest on your side, and position a rolled towel to rest your cheek on. Note that whether in the bath or a birth pool, having your partner pour water gently and rhythmically down your back can feel good, as can having an ice cube massaged in circles on your lower back. The contrast of the warm water and the cold ice provides distraction.

It was the anticipation of it. Every time a contraction was over and I could rest, my doula would repetitively pour water down my back from a little jug, and always with the same, slow rhythm. She'd stop when the wave began to build, and resume pouring once it was over, so the ritual became a kind of cue – to focus on the work when there was work to do; to welcome and relish my rest when there was rest to be had.

Sally

You may want to save your birth pool for the end, when the pressure in your pelvis and bottom is growing very intense. You can use a bath or shower before this point, and wait until the urge to immerse yourself fully is irresistible. There's often a physiological pay-off. Mind and muscles relax so completely in water once labour is very advanced, that you can almost feel the extra space opening up in your back and bottom. Labour often speeds towards its lovely conclusion from there.

A little word on pacing

As you'll learn in the next chapter, the beginning of birth needs ignoring – or at least pretend ignoring – and is best achieved by conducting a normal day. A NORMAL normal day. No setting the scene, or getting into gear. Just business as usual. Your partner going to work (he can check in mid-morning to see if you want company); meeting a friend or going for a walk; making dinner; sorting and cleaning; reading a book or writing emails; watching a film. Even ironing can be a pleasurable distraction.

In due course, and it really could be anything between a few hours and a couple of days, things will develop and your body will demand more attention. This is the time to employ comforts more actively – to put on some relaxing music, or run a bath. To pull a blanket over you in bed and doze-breathe for a bit. It's true that being active in labour can help. But avoid too much effort – marching about or squatting for example – as it's unnecessary and you'll wear yourself out. If your baby and body want you to do something, they will tell you.

You still might not be in labour – the part where your baby starts to move deeply down and through your pelvis – so pace yourself. Contractions will crank up, and even feel intense. But if you bob up in between them, if you could get yourself a drink for example, or tap out a long text, relax. Pause and allow yourself to adjust. Find the comfort that fits the feeling.

There are two reasons to avoid firing labour's starter gun. First, labour is involuntary, so lighting candles, calling doulas and creating a zone won't make the birth happen any sooner. Second, for a first birth especially, it's absolutely vital that you pace yourself – mentally, emotionally, and of course physically. Over-focusing and working too hard, too early, can use vital reserves before they're necessary.

Once you are in established labour and the feelings are progressive and propulsive, every bit of you will be involved – all your attention taken. Now is the time for your partner or doula to alter the mood to match your needs – darkening rooms, lighting candles and filling the pool.

I slept for a whole afternoon in the early stages of labour. I remember I felt really tired, so I drew the curtains, got comfy with a hot water bottle and a blanket, and drifted off. I'd surface when a wave came of course, but once it had passed, I'd doze off again. I felt expectant – but I wasn't watching myself, or wondering what was going on. I was just so relieved I'd booked a midwife to come to me, because it meant I didn't have to think or do anything until I wanted her there. I could just do what felt good, at that point. In the evening, I felt recharged. My husband made dinner, we had this funny romantic supper at the kitchen table with a candle, and about an hour later, things got much stronger, so I had a bath.

Though I was having to close my eyes and breathe

with focus, I knew it wasn't labour – because there was no change in my body. My doula had told me when the time came, I would feel my baby exerting pressure, a kind of growing weight, and as there was nothing like that, I made my husband go to bed in the spare room and rested some more, with the help of some relaxation music. At some point in the night, that big shift did come – and I had to get on my hands and knees by the side of the bed.

I started to sigh, hum and moan I think, and I guess my husband must have heard me, or peeped in. I don't know. I was just totally absorbed with the job in hand. I knew now that that was all I had to do – concentrate – and that he would take care of everything else. My midwife and doula arrived at some point after that but I couldn't say when. All I knew was if I needed the toilet, I'd find myself on the toilet – or I'd be in the shower and think, yes, this IS what I wanted. I liked the water on my back, the cold tiles on my forehead, and then suddenly, I just remember having this almighty urge to squat down – I could feel the baby pressing hard, the starting of an urge to push. My eyes were closed and all I was doing was focusing on each feeling as it came. No one said a thing... and everything felt very clear and sure. The sensation of her coming out was the clearest thing I have ever felt. I was on all fours in the bathroom, leaning forward onto a pile of soft towels someone had made me. And the next thing I knew – she was there. My baby was in my arms.

Julia

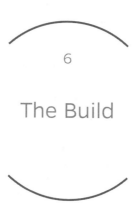

6

The Build

Bookshop shelves are full of information about childbirth. The internet too, of course. Yet useful knowledge, about how labour *feels*, is curiously hard to come by. Clinical framing – birth as a linear sequence – is everywhere. Stages of labour, cervical dilation, contractions as things you count. But these are constructions defined by measurement, from the perspective of an observer. The *lived* version – straightforward labour as it would be felt first hand – is rarely shared and frustratingly hard to find.

If you think about it, this is strange. There are seven billion people on the planet. Homo sapiens have been giving birth for 200,000 years. How is it possible for women, in the West at least, and at this hyper-informed point in history, to know and understand so little about an experience so many have gone and will go through? More bewildering still, why is it that books, courses and medical experts (most of whom will not have experienced normal labour) are the go-to authority on birth?

Given that most women will give birth to a baby, and it is a normal, universal physical function, why aren't *we* holding the wisdom about it? Why isn't insight transmitted automatically, as a shared part of female experience?

Birthing by numbers

One glaring gap in our knowledge concerns the *build* to birth. Hospital has been the predominant location for delivery for some decades. Even so, it's taken a while to understand the different ways that moving a mother mid-birth to a different space can impact on the process. It's long been realised that a change in environment can cause labour to slow. But deciding 'when' to go to hospital is another problem area, and is where tension and adrenaline begin to creep in.

When the labour ward is the destination, a huge amount of focus gets put on arrival, on the part where you are actually having the baby, as well as a number of simplistic, standard-issue indicators that are supposed to help gauge that point. It's as if hurrying to the place where you're having the baby, hastens the baby.

But there is a whole lot more to birth than the final straight. Vital physical and emotional readying needs to take place. In early birth, women enter a liminal, sensitive state and being relaxed and having no plan can help you settle into this.

As Dr Rachel Reed explains:

Labour is basically the process by which a baby moves from the inside of a woman to the outside of a woman. Sounds simple, but it is incredibly complex and involves a complicated interplay of physiological, psychological and emotional factors. Women's experience of labour often involves a sense of separation from the external world, focusing within, and becoming immersed in the act of giving birth. The hormones released during birth support this 'altered state of consciousness' (see the work of Sarah Buckley). During early labour the woman is beginning to move into this birthing state.

This move *into* the birthing state is as important as the birthing state itself and needs respecting – a phase of labour, but a key part of birth as a whole. The active phase of labour is involuntary, highly coordinated and, for the body to reach that tipping point, some elaborate groundwork (i.e. early labour) is first required. The cervix needs to soften and give (the opposite of what it's been doing for nine months), the baby needs to sink deeper into the pelvis, the uterus needs to get into gear, and the mother herself needs to feel completely comfortable and deeply safe. Without this as a foundation, her body can't commit to its course.

The forgotten knowledge

Few women arrive at full term with a realistic expectation or proper understanding of this run-up to birth – the time it can take for example, or the support that's needed to help them recognise it, relax into it and accept it as necessary. As a result, there's uncertainty. This leads to impatience and anxiety, and a vast number of couples head for hospital before labour has really begun.

Imagine how different things will be if you are having your baby at home. Imagine how it will feel *not* having to make that decision. There being no destination to reach; no worry about discomfort en route; no fear about being admitted or not.

'A mother at home doesn't need to concern herself with "when to go to hospital", says Dr Rachel Reed. 'And her midwife can (should) attend based on when the woman needs her… not when she meets particular criteria.'

Having a baby at home restores natural flow and continuity. What you want to have happen *happens*, based on your body's instructive cues rather than a pre-emptive assessment of how you're doing. The build may be hours, it may be days. But in your own space, where you're in charge and can respond naturally to what your body's doing, time is unimportant. Distraction is easy. Normal life is happily and conveniently to hand and helps you to manage expectations and conserve energy while your body is getting ready. Of course, even if you do need to go to hospital for the birth for some reason, this 'forgotten knowledge' can still improve your experience of birth in hospital, by giving you the confidence to stay at home for longer and not to rush in.

As recently as the 1960s, when birth at home was still commonplace, there would have been a collective, confident grasp of labour's build. Firstly, women would have witnessed it many times. Secondly, when it was your turn, you would have had support. When contractions began, a first-time mother would have had her own mother nearby, or an aunt or neighbour, normalising everything and showing her the way.

There'd have been no labelling as such, or discussion about 'stages'. Women with experience knew early labour wasn't medically significant and would have helped the mother to be resourceful, self-reliant and to manage how she felt. They'd have made some tea or hung out a wash. They'd have done the day as normal while it didn't look or feel like labour and communicated a reassuring message: 'this isn't it yet, but all is as it should be.'

I had my first baby at home in 1952 and went on to have four more at home too. I can remember when it started even now, and the first thing I did was call my mum. I had to go to a phonebox as we didn't have a phone at home then, and she came round. She didn't rush round, because there was no reason to. I remember she just turned up, took off her coat, got settled in and looked after me. She knew I liked to read, so she got me to sit in an armchair and read my book. I remember the pains hurting, but my mum just carried on – doing a bit of cleaning I think, or maybe she peeled some potatoes. And I remember thinking oh well, it's just normal. I just got on with it. That was all day, and then that night she made me a bed up in the front room and got me comfortable. She stayed that night and didn't call the midwife until the next afternoon – until it was time.

Edie Purdue, age 84

If you are having your baby at home, copy Edie! You could try to find three women who've had positive birth experiences at home, and ask them how the build-up felt for them. Mother-to-mother guidance is invaluable. Avoid having a fixed idea about how things may start, or even any kind of plan, as just as we all get hungry and tired at different times and in different ways, birth's first feelings vary too – both in timeframe and experience. Instead get familiar with what to expect more generally, along with some advance ideas on how to pace yourself, and on the day you'll be ready to relax.

I had a long night of spaced contractions at the start of my birth, and then in the morning things started to feel very strong. Regular too. I was needing to lean now, and breathe hard, although in the rests I felt normal. I was alone at home with my partner, and I think if we'd not done the homework – certainly if we'd not planned a home birth, we'd have thought I was in labour.

Luckily for me, I had a friend who'd had three babies at home and called her. Just before she answered, I realised that if I could call her, I probably wasn't in labour. Even so it was lovely to speak to her, and she confirmed just that. Both she and my midwife had said that I'd recognise labour because it was extremely, extremely intense. That it would demand total concentration, even in the rests. I remember my friend saying I wouldn't want or be able to watch telly for example, or make a sandwich. That I just wouldn't want to do anything but breathe deeply, moan a bit and close my eyes – and that until I was feeling that way, to distract myself or relax as best I could.

'Brilliant!' my friend said. 'You're doing amazing! Go and have a bath'. My goodness, her advice really saved me some energy – emotionally and physically. We were just about to blow the pool up, to start setting everything up and get the midwife over. Now instead, I had that bath, then went for a rest in bed while my husband took the dog for a walk. I rested all afternoon in fact and he made a shepherd's pie for dinner. Then around 6pm, I felt this huge shift in intensity. I got it now – that it changes, and then changes again, that the feelings grow and deepen at regular intervals and all without me doing anything. It all made sense and the funniest thing of all, I felt like I knew exactly what to do. The midwife came round at about seven and my baby was born just before midnight.

Karen

Waiting

In recent years, due dates seem to have become tripwires. The weeks running up to a baby's arrival were once filled with joy, but now they can be fraught with stress. A side-effect of continuous maternity care as it's currently delivered is an emphasis on dates and measurement, such that even when a mother is well, her pregnancy healthy and she is fully familiar with the facts (term is a 37 to 42 week window not a specific date), it's easy to feel anxious. Women can feel cornered and even coerced into encouraging labour with sweeps, booking induction dates and even induction itself.

When you're having your baby at home, it's different. On your own territory, deadlines and dictates can be seen for what they are – guidelines. Self-trust will be high and the sense of personal responsibility developed through pregnancy and preparing will help you feel empowered. So if 42 weeks does swing into sight, approach it positively. Talk to your midwife. Weigh up the risks of waiting with the risks of induction. And make decisions that feel right for you. This is what Eden did.

I had planned to have my baby at home. When I reached my 40-week appointment, I decided to get ahead of the game and ask my midwife what their usual procedure is when a woman passes her 'due date'. At this point I was informed that they 'do not allow women to go past 40+12' and would book me in for an induction by this time. I decided to politely challenge the language 'allow women', which my midwife rephrased as 'advise' and explained that a woman can choose to decline induction, but this would be a conversation they would have with a doctor at the hospital. I took a leaflet about their pessary induction procedure and after a lot of independent research of our own, made an informed decision with my partner that this form of induction would not be for us. Shortly after my 41-week appointment, my partner and I attended the hospital to meet with a doctor to discuss declining an induction offer. For the first time in my whole pregnancy my blood pressure was really high, as I naturally started to feel anxious due to the language being used by care providers for deciding to take a course of action outside of the recommendations. The doctor was focused on describing the risk of going past 42 weeks to us. However, it was clear that absolute and relative risks were being blurred, while generalised statistics were being used giving a very inaccurate picture. We were aware of women who had gone on to have natural births at 42 weeks and even 44 weeks and having healthy babies, so made an informed decision to again decline induction.

On a side note, you are still entitled to midwife care at home post-42 weeks, and if a healthcare professional suggests otherwise remind them that it is the NHS's responsibility to provide you with a midwife at home, and at whatever point, if that is your request.

Awaiting is harder than waiting – because there are unknowns attached. That's just the way of it. Be a journeywoman. Keep your hand on the tiller and be ready to steady yourself. Get excited, feel expectant – cherish this precious, threshold time in the knowledge that if your body went to the effort to grow a baby, it has a plan for letting it out.

'The induction of labour poses a real threat to a woman's chance of giving birth to her baby by herself' says midwife, author and researcher Sara Wickham. 'So unless there is a good medical reason to start intervention, don't be robbed. You're going to feel soft and sensitive, a strange sort of heightening in these last few days and weeks – so experience the wonder of that. Clean, sort, swim, read, knit, cook. Let your body go about its business and let the build to take its course. When your baby gives the cue, a straightforward labour is more likely.'

Your baby is having ideas

The signal that things are beginning was described to me by my wonderful doula as 'Your baby is having ideas'. For something so fuzzy, it is spot-on precise, for this is just how it feels. Tightenings, grumblings, cramps and crampy-waves, pressure in your groin, the mucus plug (show). All are proof that your body is bang on track. Mild contractions that stop and start may also be felt. Feel secretly pleased, stay beautifully patient and be mindful of two things: 1. it can go on for some days, and 2. business as usual.

The first room

Until the real business of labour begins – when the cervix progressively pulls up over the baby's head – see yourself as being in the 'first room'. This is an easier and more helpful way to visualise what your body is doing at this point, as terms like 'latent labour' or 'early labour' can be confusing.

It can be a wearing experience to approach birth as an ever-strengthening sequence, measuring it from the first contraction that costs you. And for first-time mums especially, this can make things feel protracted. But seeing this first phase as an anteroom – a separate place from labour where the body is readying and contractions still coordinating –will help you to position and pace yourself, to settle into it and relax.

It will be easy to dismiss cramping, or even irregular waves, but as soon as there is a marked rise-peak-recede to the sensations, and contractions are causing you to pause and lean, it's tempting to get into gear and call it labour.

When a home birth is planned, plenty of couples start burning candles, or close the curtains and create a zone. But using the L-word before it's time may set the stage too early. All that watching yourself equates to a kind of holding your breath. By circling on balls, keeping partners home and calling doulas, you've announced 'get set, GO!' and it can be hard to go back on that and recover precious energy.

A more productive approach is to save that focus for when the feelings are non-negotiable – for when you enter the second room – labour – and there is no choice but to concentrate. Labour's powerful and repeating rhythm will be unwaveringly intense and absorbing. There's a huge shift to the sensations – a shove forward that you cannot miss. So put that contraction app away and wait for when the change becomes obvious.

Get comfortable. Breathe the waves when they come; place a hot water bottle where it hits the spot. But whether it's low down cramps or contractions you're closing your eyes for, be patient. If you surface at the end of each wave and willingly reengage with whoever or whatever's around you, you're still in the first room. Distract yourself, with as much normal life as you can manage. Like Emma, who baked a birthday cake. Or Eleanor, who took a slow walk to the high street to get a picture framed. Or Lindsay, who went for a pub lunch and, though she had to stand when a wave came, wouldn't leave until she'd got her sticky toffee pudding. And finally Lucy, who weeded her garden in the winter sun all the while there was available light.

Normal is what you would be doing if your belly wasn't up to stuff. Which makes a 7am march round the park to encourage things an error. Which means partners staying at home may be something to rethink. In fact, persuading partners to be normal can be the hardest bit! They may feel a need to act. Or you feel – or think you feel – anxious. But remember the first room. If what you're feeling are crampy waves, you're not having a baby any time soon. Though it may be a comfort to have your other half there at breakfast, if nothing much has changed by teatime you'll be driving each other round the bend, wondering if something is wrong. But nothing is wrong. You just aren't in labour yet.

So, instead of self-assessing, or trying to get things going, pitch your response prudently and relax. Breathe slowly as a wave washes through, then snuggle back under a blanket and watch your film. Or swing your hips and sigh it out, before carrying on that hands and knees wash of the kitchen floor. Or, if it's night time, drift back to sleep. Make it business as usual until you can't anymore and you've got yourself a benchmark. When you no longer want to look up, when the contractions take you deep inside and it just feels better to stay there, your baby's no longer just having ideas. They are probably on their way.

Second and subsequent births

Second and subsequent labours can be quicker than first labours, though not always. There'll still likely be a build, a period where the body is preparing. For some it will be hardly noticeable, a kind of heavy, dragging feeling. Others might feel proper contractions for a few consecutive evenings, which stop when they go to sleep. Or you might have a whole day of crampy waves that then suddenly intensify. The difference the second time around is that when things do accelerate, they usually do so suddenly and then established labour is often short from there; at home, where everything is in place and the mother can just relax into it, it may even be just an hour or two.

The good news is that when things do gather pace, at home the response is simple. Just head for your bedroom, or a comfortable space where you feel safe and able to concentrate. There is no stress, you have everything you need and if you feel change with every wave, it would be a good idea to call your midwife and tell her to come promptly. The best benchmark will be your toddler or older children. All the while you can tend to them, do, because this is a sure sign that you aren't in labour yet. If you can read a story, or make the tea, carry on as normal (hot water bottles can help, or pausing to lean and breathe) and then at some point, you will feel that shift in intensity, a point when now you can't manage your child and the contractions need more focus. Call on your supporters to take care of the children, then head for your safe space. Labour is beginning.

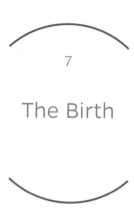

7

The Birth

Something different happens when your body agrees to let go of the baby. There is an almighty shift in gear. Your body takes over and the birth proceeds on autopilot. Established labour feels highly organised and, when conditions are conducive, is usually productive and predictable. In your own home it can be especially efficient, as there is no unnecessary discomfort or disturbance to distract you, and your body has its best chance to function optimally.

The second room

Active labour isn't a stage you reach; it is a state you *enter*. It is so different in experience to the build, it will feel like you've entered a whole new room. Ordinary awareness of time and what's around you drops away, and all you can and *want* to do is focus on the feelings, which will be powerful, urgent and clear.

The rests between contractions demand total attention too. Once you're in labour, you'll probably close your eyes and keep them closed, in order to draw what you need from them. There's no bobbing up in the breaks, or deciding on something, like getting yourself a drink or sending a text. And there is usually next to no desire to engage with who or what is around you. During contractions, you'll likely want to hang off or lean forward on something, or even lie on your side, as now that there's growing pressure, unsupported standing can feel too much. In the vast majority of labours, contractions are extremely intense, very regular and reliably rhythmic. They'll also be good and long, lasting about 10 or 12 slow, deep breaths.

> Not everyone steps into this second room. For whatever reason, some women never get into the zone – that drifty place where the world feels far away. There'll always be a number of mothers who, for personal reasons, remain alert thoughout labour and that's because they need to. To feel safe, some people maintain some self-vigilance, so if this resonates with you, be aware that your own private space, which you can control, will be more important than ever. So long as comfort and loving care are provided (supporters shouldn't take self-awareness as licence to engage), your body will get on with it anyway, so be as you wish to be. Trust that your body will labour in the way it wants to.

Protect the flow

Your body has taken a huge and sensitive step and, to open successfully, is now releasing high levels of oxytocin, the hormone that fires contractions, drives labour and needs privacy, safety and quiet to flow.

The need to retreat will feel natural and necessary – your

body is expressing it's now pressing need to be protected – and you'll probably find yourself drawn to the quietest, smallest space in the house, like a back bedroom or bathroom. The seclusion aids concentration and helps you to immerse yourself in the way your body requires. You can't sleep and think all at once, and birth is the same. The active phase of labour insists on full focus, so wait for it to feel that way and if nothing and no one is disturbing you, you'll feel compelled to respond.

Doula and Alexander Technique teacher Ilana Machover says:

> *The mother cannot directly control her autonomous nervous system or her hormonal balance and any attempt to do this will be self-defeating. The woman does not 'do' anything to give birth: the dilation of the cervix happens by itself, and all she needs to 'do' is to allow the process to proceed. With each contraction, she should just move in a relaxed way, agree to accept the pain, and help herself to cope with it.*

Privacy provides safety. Now that your body has committed to its course, labour's engine room, the hypothalamus, is bent on getting the job done in order to limit this period of vulnerability for you and your baby to as short a time as possible. Feeling observed and assessed can create performance pressure and arouse expectation. This triggers adrenaline, which can slow labour down. But when self-awareness evaporates, your body has its fullest chance of doing what it needs to do, in the way it needs to do it – with the result that birth is often straightforward.

Unlike the initial stages – where I found that I had to deliberately focus through contractions – labour itself felt much simpler. I felt very safe and protected and became completely drawn into myself, to the point where I wasn't thinking anymore and had much less awareness or care about what was going on around me.

In this state, things took on a clarity and all the layers of planning, expectation and anticipation dropped away. I had a strong sense that things were working as they should, so much so that it became completely obvious to me that my body would know how to give birth.

I felt I could almost see what was happening as each stage progressed, as if I had an internal map of my body in my mind's eye. Again this wasn't a conscious thought, but more of a general 'knowing'. I had originally intended to go into hospital; however the thought of moving, let alone going out in public and getting into a car, felt completely unnecessary and even absurd. I realised then that the part of me that had taken over from my usual, more socially-conforming self, was not going to be moved anywhere. This is why I ended up experiencing a wonderful, if slightly unexpected, home birth.

What helped me to feel completely safe and secure was having my doula and my husband there, and also the autonomy I felt by being in my own home. I was with people I could put my full trust in. Because of this, I was able to stop thinking and relax – knowing I had people who would 'hold the fort' for me and protect the space and privacy I had carved out around me.

Emily

Support

When your partner and/or doula sees this shift in your behaviour, they can soften and adapt your surroundings and quietly start to get things organised – like inflating and half-filling a birth pool or informing your midwife. Until this point, even if contractions have been testing, keep things as normal as possible, as creating a birth 'cave' before you are in proper labour can be counter-productive. Remember labour is involuntary. You can't make yourself labour any more than you can make yourself sleep.

Once things are underway, however, those supporting you can lower lights or darken the room completely. Candles in the bathroom or fairylights in your bedroom can be a good way to create a tranquil mood, and if you were wanting to use meditation or hypnobirthing tracks, now would be the time to introduce them.

Hot water bottles can be deftly refilled, lavender on a handkerchief quietly recharged. The trick is for supporters to attune to how you feel and what might help without directly engaging you – by being unobtrusive, observant and responding to your needs as they arise: for example covering you with a warm blanket or holding an ice-cold flannel on your forehead if you're hot; or if you're on your knees, providing cushions for support. You're not 'open for business', so a long, cold drink of water with a straw just needs producing; a warm bath can be run. A piece of cold clementine can be offered without comment.

Crucially, anyone caring for you needs to avoid 'coaching' or 'rescuing' you. 'One cannot actively help a woman to give birth. The goal is to avoid disturbing her unnecessarily,' says obstetrician Michel Odent, and if a labour is progressing normally, this advice needs heeding if it's to continue to do so. You may be moaning, sighing, sometimes even struggling, but that doesn't automatically equate to distress. If supporters step in with the assumption that you're overwhelmed, more harm than good may be done. It can make a mother hesitant and unsure to think that others are anxious on her behalf and the natural endorphin-supported confidence that flows from a physiological labour can get knocked.

But what if you do get despondent? Labours that take an unexpected turn will be looked at in the next chapter. But demoralising dips are quite common and occur in almost all labours, so if a big swell comes and you feel in need of a boost, reach out. Close contact can work wonders. A cuddle in bed with your partner, perhaps, or leaning against your doula and rocking together. Do so through a few contractions, and before long you'll feel steady, comfortable and equanimity will be restored.

Calling your midwife

You may have already called your midwife when things first began. But the point at which you *need* her to come is different and a question for you to feel rather than decide. Some women want time to find their way and enjoy the privacy and uninterrupted focus that comes with a period of time by themselves. Others like to have a midwife as soon as labour gets strong and established. The suggestion midwives make is this: 'You'll know when you need me,' so make that your guide, remembering that it is your choice entirely as to when you are attended.

If it is your first baby, there'll likely be some hours before your baby's arrival, so you have time. If it is a second or subsequent birth, babies tend to come quite quickly from the point where labour intensifies, so be aware that it might be helpful to be on your midwife's radar, and have your partner notify her when things ramp up a gear.

Once you are in active labour, the midwife stays. She has routine checks to carry out, but these are not obligatory and decisions about what is checked, how often you are checked or if you even want checking at all are entirely up to you. Basic observations include your temperature, blood pressure, pulse, the position and descent of the baby as well as any changes in the colour of the waters or blood loss. Hospital guidelines usually recommend a foetal heart rate check every 15 minutes once the mother is in established labour, and every 5 minutes when she is pushing, so consider whether this is OK for you or if you would prefer it less frequently. An electronic sonicaid is the usual method used for listening in, but some find its crackle and hiss unsettling, in which case a handheld pinard is an alternative option. Aside from the checks, your midwife will mostly stay out of your way unless you request otherwise. She may sit at your kitchen table, writing up her notes, or listen from a hidden vantage point, like the landing.

I had no awareness of my midwife for most of my labour. I knew she was close – and that felt nice. Safe. But I loved the feeling of being completely unselfconscious and free, of her not watching me as I laboured, waiting for things to happen. After the birth, my husband told me she'd spent most of the time sitting on the floor in the spare bedroom, with a cup of tea on her lap.

Becky

When your baby's arrival is close, a second midwife is called to assist. A new person entering your space at this sensitive moment can feel disturbing, so if you don't want her in the room or simply want her to stay out of view until you are actually delivering, make that clear in your birth preferences and/or through discussions beforehand.

Coping

Follow your body's cues, assume positions that feel good and find a space that's comfortable. Draw on the support of those caring for you, and remember that intensifying contractions are something to welcome – what you want and need for the baby to be born.

Intense is great. But more intense is better than that. And more intense still is the signal to find yourself and what is happening amazing – certainly for your partner to give you a big kiss of encouragement. Because your baby is coming.

There's conductivity now. Easy power. Plug into that charge and you'll find the repeating rhythm holds you. There's a tendency to think that labour gets harder the further it goes. But in a normal labour, in birth-friendly conditions, it often feels the opposite. Like the wind is at your back. There's certainty to the sensations, an unmissable sense that you're moving towards your baby.

Breathe deeply, rock from foot to foot, sit on the loo or lean forward on a pile of pillows. Hang off your headboard, or sink into your partner's chest and feel held. Sing a long, loud note, and when it feels irresistible not to, sink into your birth pool. In between the work, stay focused on your breathing. Notice its rhythmic flow – the way it's always there for you, keeping you and your baby safe. And use your rests to relax – to loosen and let go of your whole body.

With Elias I woke in the night and couldn't sleep. After a while lying on the sofa my waters broke. I walked around the flat a bit and then it started hurting and it was very uncomfortable. This was a few hours after the waters broke. Things got more intense with contractions getting stronger and closer. I spent some undefined time in the bath and when I emerged from it, it was day! At this point the labour changed and I felt the urge to push. There was a lot of standing with open legs and squatting. Then after final pushes Elias slid out. It had taken 12 hours. Most of it is a blur. With Mei, my second child, it was much faster. I woke and within 15 minutes, I knew the baby was moving down. There was no build bit – it was intense and progressive from the beginning and the whole thing took three hours. Again I have a physical memory of Mei sliding out. I think the main things that made the home birth for me were: being in a familiar environment; knowing the important people and trusting them and when it was all done we were already at home. Most of all though it was that after the birth and before the placenta my husband and I got to spend the first moments of our children's lives on the outside together in peace and quiet. No interruptions, no unfamiliar sounds and smells, no thinking about the journey home or the night in hospital. I don't hate hospital but it's where you go when you're ill. Giving birth is more like running a (half) marathon at the end of which you meet the love of your life and get married. You don't want to end that day at hospital, but at home where you can rest and process the event.

Sarah

If a moment comes when it feels too hard, and your mind and body feel tense and resistant, connect to your purpose. Remind yourself of what you're engaged in: THE MOST MAGNIFICENT EVENT OF YOUR LIFE. Of course it feels huge. Breathe frankincense oil on a handkerchief to ground yourself and try repeating an affirmation:

I can do this
I AM doing this

How do I know labour is progressing?

Women don't often hear this, but the building sensation of your baby nudging, bearing, dropping and drawing lower is extremely marked. There is nothing clearer in all the world than a baby making its way down and through your pelvis, and when you tune into that feeling, labour starts to make good physical sense.

It was like a burrowing feeling. – Eleanor

You can feel your bottom spreading. – Isla

It's a feeling of filling up – a growing heaviness, like when you're constipated. – Katy

It's just different – deeper, wider, fuller – once the baby is moving down. There's a lot of pressure. – Meredith

Only you can feel the changes inside your body, which makes you the expert on whether things are progressing. What greater guide could there be than the mother whose body is experiencing it?

Along with building pressure in your vagina and bottom, the peaks of the contractions will feel growingly intense. The urge to make louder moans to match the wave may also feel irresistible, as releasing the jaw automatically releases the pelvic floor, providing room and relief. You may feel trembly for a period, and grow hot – pull-your-clothes-off hot – because your body is working incredibly hard. In very advanced labour, you feel like you need to poo. This is the baby's head pressing on and moving past your rectum.

If you are feeling regular internal changes, you are very, very, very likely to be progressing, so take comfort from that.

Let it embolden you and take you forward, as there's nothing like knowing you're getting there to reinforce your focus. Never fear that you're not up to it, or that you haven't the strength or stamina. Successful birth isn't left to the individual – the continuation of the human race depends on it. You are designed to cope, and will cope, like millions of mothers have before you.

The medical yardstick measures labour as beginning when the cervix has dilated to 4cm. But my doula sense tells me that labour's give-point in fact varies from mother to mother. It is an emotional as well as a physical juncture and though it may well be 4cm for some, it could be 7cm for others and, in cases where babies have some turning to do, maybe even at the very last. The point is, labour is not about a magical millimetre, which is why vaginal exams, the routine way of measuring whether you are progressing, aren't the best guide.

Your midwife will offer you a vaginal examination when she arrives, and once you are in established labour again every four hours, but if you can feel changes for yourself, and feel encouraged by that, you might want to consider what it will add. Internal exams are not a reliable indicator of how birth will progress and they can put the focus back on the clock. Apart from feeling invasive at this sensitive point, for it to be performed you'll be required to lie on your back, albeit very briefly. Besides this, you're awaiting a 'result' – the measure of how you are doing and the rationalising that results (you inevitably do the maths), which can 'bring you to your senses' and affect oxytocin flow. Four cm and you're demoralised. Ten cm and there's a drum roll. No news is good news, my doula always said, so be wary of the idea that a number presents an incentive. However, exams may be useful when a decision needs making – for example if labour has been overly long and wearing and you're thinking of transferring to hospital.

Remember that it is entirely up to you if you wish to consent to internal exams – no one can insist on them.

The baby arrives

Imagine pulling a polo neck jumper over your head – how easily it slides when it reaches your ears. In the last stage of opening, where the last of the cervix is slipping over the baby's head, there is a similar momentum, and it can feel crashy and climactic.

In this transitional phase, mothers often become agitated, sometimes saying things like, 'I can't do this', or 'I don't want a baby anymore'. The fear is physiological, triggered by the necessary release of adrenaline that carries women past this peak-point and on to the birth of the baby. So it's important that it's not disturbed, for example by people jumping in to reassure you, or doing stuff to lift you out of it.

It soon passes, and as the baby starts to make its way down the birth canal, contractions slow and space, giving mothers a much-needed rest. Soon after, minutes if it is a second birth, an hour or more if it's the first – the baby's head meets the pelvic floor and the pushy feelings you will already have been experiencing start to get expulsive.

> My midwife said the perfect thing when the moment came to push. 'Do nothing'. It probably sounds strange, but it was so helpful as it helped me to realise that the force of it all is just happening anyway, and all you're really doing is going along with it.
>
> Simone

At home, midwives tend to be hands-off when it comes to delivery and allow the baby to birth itself. You'll naturally find a position that feels right – a half kneel, or leaning forward on your sofa – and now all there is to do is go with it. Trust your body completely. Some women like a hot flannel being pressed on their perineum at this point, as it can be soothing. Talk to your midwife beforehand about what you might want, and if you're clear you don't want any touching or obvious delivering of your baby at all, have it recorded in your notes so that all the midwives in your team are aware of your wishes.

I remember the moment where I felt a significant change in the progress of my labour. A definite 'ramping up' inside of me. My body actually spoke to me, almost a 'Here we go girl, get ready to focus' and no matter how much mental preparation I'd done it did shake me.

I remember asking my doula if I could 'take my knickers off now' and she of course said, 'whatever you need to do'. At that moment little did I know I was only 45 minutes away from my baby arriving. Time seemed to stand still almost and I went 'into myself'. Without thinking I went into the lounge (my dark quiet place) and leant on my birth ball by my sofa. I just felt the most comfortable that way and I was aware of these small, long, low grunts coming out of my mouth with every contraction.

I felt calm and the world seemed distant, my mind had shrunk to only the task in hand. My eyes were shut, I tried to visualise rose petals slowly blossoming and my internal voice was telling me to remain calm; the calmer I am, I thought, the more relaxed I am, and the quicker the baby will be here. I felt focused, and centred. Safe and free. I didn't allow anyone to 'perform any checks', I felt too protective of my body and what it was doing. After 20 minutes or so (I wasn't looking at the time, but that is what I was told) I could literally feel the lips of

*my vagina peeling back, opening up at a fast pace. My
body had completely taken over, the process seemed to
accelerate rapidly and I had no control over what it
was doing. Part of me was in awe and part in shock
at just how strong my body was. I was completely
alive with deeply purposeful feelings. It felt right, and
as long as I let go I felt sure things would continue to
go well. As the contractions got stronger they'd moved
from my stomach to my pelvic area and I knew I was
close. I then felt such a tremendous pressure building
between my legs that just as I thought 'I can't take
this anymore', I'm stretched to the max, out my baby
rocketed into the room. The relief afterwards is so
sweet. It was almost as if I'd been hypnotised, as once
my baby was out, it's like I was instantly 'back in the
room'. I felt deeply emotional and thankful that I'd
trusted my body and grateful that my baby had come
to me safely in such a truly amazing and memorable
way. My birthing experience literally shook me to my
core and has had a profoundly positive and lasting
effect on my whole life.*

Suzy

First moments

Babies may have been emerging for millennia, but those first
moments are never anything less than extraordinary. Your
midwife passes you your baby, or if you're in the pool, helps
you to gather him or her on to your chest. Then you just take
your time, taking your baby in. There's no rush. No change.
You're made warm and comfortable, the cord continues to
connect you and you can relax and absorb the startling fact
that your baby is here.

The womb to world shift is seismic for a newborn, and

what they want is enough warm, calm quiet to find what they need. You.

Warm, calm quiet is exactly what you need too, as once your baby is born, the hormone oxytocin has to peak so that a last few contractions can safely birth the placenta.

Make sure partners are aware of this, and that there is no uprush of activity – for example calls to family or the taking of photos – as the birth is still not complete and needs the same conditions you had in labour.

You can deliver the placenta in the pool if you used one, or your partner can have a cosy nest of blankets, towels and a pillow pre-prepared. Lie on your side, cuddle your baby, and rest.

It can take up to an hour for the placenta to deliver naturally, and if you start to feel a growing heaviness in your vagina, some gravity might feel helpful. Remember that self-consciousness inhibits oxytocin, so if you feel in any way on view, ask for privacy. With sufficient protection, the placenta usually arrives of its own accord.

If it doesn't, your midwife can manage the delivery by giving you an injection. The use of drugs for the third stage may be specific to your local area. Syntocinon is the most common, unless there is excessive bleeding, in which case a combination of syntocinon (to create contractions) and ergometrine (to stop bleeding) is used. All drugs can cause nausea, dizziness and vomiting, but those with ergometrine tend to cause it more, so make sure to have a conversation with your midwives in advance about your preferences, so that they're recorded in your notes.

Important checks will be carried out on you and baby after the baby is born to ensure both of you are doing well and there are no concerns. But unless there is a clear problem, this shouldn't mean your time with your new baby is disturbed.

Make sure that your midwife knows that you want routine checks to be delayed to give you undisturbed time with your baby.

After the placenta is delivered, the midwife will check for perineal damage and suture (stitch) if needs be. A local anaesthetic is administered, but breathing lavender from a handkerchief can also help with the discomfort, as well as gas and air if it's available. The midwife or your partner can sort you some knickers and a thick sanitary pad, help you on with a clean nightdress or T-shirt and then get you into bed with your baby. And that's it! Time for tea and toast and a cuddle.

The brilliant thing about giving birth at home is the way you can't help but spill into the experience, especially second time round. It's like a normal day, only everything becomes more vibrant and raw somehow. It's like you step right into the heart of life and truly feel what it all means. You're at home – right at the centre of your home. Your family and chosen support begin to gather and there is a feeling of love and collaboration. It's unspoken to a degree and things seem to fall into place the way they should – it feels natural.

Someone sweeps the kitchen floor and tidies away the dishes from supper; someone runs a bath and a close friend arrives to cuddle your toddler, towels and sheets appear and the room fills with the scent of lavender from your garden. You are home, really home. Everything swells with the anticipation of the welcoming.

A moment comes when you feel the light in your eyes turns inward – to your baby. In the quiet, soft and dark of your own room – the space where your baby first took hold inside you – you connect with her and a profound silent meeting takes place. It is just you and her. Even the sounds from your own mouth seem far away and incidental as, together in unspoken harmony, you work and work. You fill with a strange familiar peace – as if you've always known this moment would come. It feels perfectly right and with that comfort and acceptance comes the sensation of a real and exquisite pleasure as your baby descends, or rather seems to float her way through you, away from you and towards you all at once. She is like a feather brushing you from within and there is a kind of whispering back and forth as you guide each other towards encounter. At the moment of birth there is a sudden crescendo as you finally feel the hard edge of her physical being. For that moment you are suspended in time and motion. Everything is about that burning delight – you are all purpose and potential as you bring your baby into the air.

Eilidh

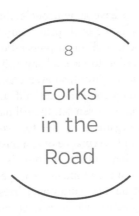

8

Forks
in the
Road

Birth at home isn't always straightforward. As with a hospital birth, there may be issues before labour, during labour, or after labour. A fork in the road won't always mean you'll need to change plan and have your baby in hospital. In the case of an advance issue, some research, an informed choice and a reset might be all that's needed. But if a complication arises that requires medical management, resist seeing it as a disaster or letting disappointment dominate.

Like all natural life events, birth is unpredictable. All we can do is set things up, prepare to the best of our ability and then, if the birth veers from the path we planned, take a philosophical step back and loosen our attachment to it. In her piece in *Midwifery Today*, 'Thoughts on Homebirth Transfer', New York-based doula Mary Esther Molloy describes one mother's mindset: 'She created an open space from which to enter birth… she was passionate about what she wanted, but there was ease about the birth itself.'

When there's a plan to have a baby at home, it's easy to become bound to the idea. Interruptions are often viewed in binary terms: things have 'gone wrong' rather than right. This may be because a home birth plan requires a level of deep personal investment – all birth preparation should include this – but the decision to have a baby at home demands an explicit commitment upfront, so even considering deviation from the imagined outcome may feel difficult.

Strong intention has been set; there'll have been a fair bit of planning and organisation. But this is only a resource. The self-reliance and acceptance of responsibility that comes with preparing to have a baby at home is a continuum and won't just desert you the moment a change of plan becomes necessary. You will be able to draw on it, irrespective of setting or outcome. In practice, when women end up needing to transfer they often feel positive and unregretful about their original plan to birth at home, and in most cases return to it undeterred for subsequent pregnancies. Perhaps this is because the inbuilt positives, like taking charge and expecting to be heard and respected by caregivers, hold firm, whatever path birth takes.

I was transferred to hospital for the birth of my first daughter because I started bleeding more than normal during labour. The transfer was very smooth, in an ambulance without a rush, and the midwife was very supportive. Once in hospital the birth continued to be straightforward, with no complications. But we were glad we went in – it felt right given the increased risk. It was a hypnobirthing affirmation that helped me adjust most I think. It said: 'My birth will happen in its own way, in its own time'. So I kept thinking that. I also 'knew' instinctively my baby was OK. And of course the midwife kept monitoring too. There was never a sense of danger, but a feeling that it was the way it was supposed to be. My husband was really calm too. He had done the hypnobirthing course with me and knew how important it was to stay calm. I also had no fear and no sense of failure for going to hospital. I had prepared myself. I knew 45% of first home births end up in hospital. And there was no medical intervention, so everything was as nature intended it to be. It was an amazing experience even though we had to go to hospital. I had my second daughter at home three weeks ago. We decided to still plan a home birth as our first experience was very positive. The only downside was that it took many consultant appointments to get signed off for a home birth this time round. Although my pregnancy was low risk, they were cautious to 'allow' me a home birth because of the history.

Astrid

A level of looseness around planning birth at home and a proper understanding of the factual realities isn't just important on an individual level. It's crucial for society full stop. It is embarrassing, and even sinister, that in an era when women presume an equal chance, proper choice and the basic right to determine their own lives, they are incapacitated in their choices around birth due to disinformation.

If consumers were being as openly and actively disadvantaged as women are with their plans for birth, there'd be a watchdog on the case. But Ofbirth has yet to be formed. In the meantime, we must detonate the myths for ourselves and up there, ripe for explosion, is the notion that when things go wrong in a home birth, it is vastly more dangerous than when things go wrong in hospital.

While no one much thinks about the very great likelihood of birth becoming long and complicated in an obstetric setting, what-ifs about home birth abound. In fact it's this baseless speculation that puts huge numbers of women off having a baby at home without further question, the general consensus being that a problem at home represents disproportionately more risk than the same problem in hospital.

This isn't true. Urgent emergencies are extremely rare, and in the exact same way as they would on a labour ward or birth centre, competent, vigilant midwives are skilled, trained, and fully equipped to foresee, manage and resolve unexpected eventualities. Where a situation is beyond a midwife's remit, timely transfer is arranged, with measures in place to ensure maximum safety for you and your baby. 'The things that go wrong in the majority of cases, particularly with first babies, do so slowly or with plenty of warning so that they have time to make the transfer,' explains consultant obstetrician Rick Porter of Wiltshire Healthcare Trust.

It's true that home birth transfer rates are substantial: 21% overall according to the 2011 Birthplace in England study. But these rates are not an indicator of adverse outcomes. The research found that the incidence of poor perinatal outcomes is still low in home birth, as it is in all birth settings, and that planned home birth gave low-risk women a significantly greater chance of a normal birth. Despite the transfer rate, low-risk women who had planned to birth at home were significantly less likely than those with a planned birth in obstetric units to have an instrumental or operative delivery or to receive medical intervention such as augmentation, epidural or episiotomy.

And yet, if a woman tells a tale of her home birth transfer, it will be met with an intake of breath, and an assumption that the situation was a life-or-death emergency. If she described the same scenario in hospital, for example an increase in foetal heart rate, or a request for an epidural, the response might be a concerned look.

A mindful rehearsal of plan B is a useful and grounding counterbalance to the more hysterical end of all this home birth mythology, as is a back-up hospital bag, packed with homey comforts and tucked away in a cupboard. No-notice childcare arrangements can be put in place if it is a second or subsequent birth.

Address and discuss contingencies openly with your midwife, and let the issues breathe. Think through how you'd feel about a caesarean and have your first preferences, for example gentle practices like delayed cord clamping, spelled out in a back-up birth plan.

The facts of home birth need an honest airing – in advance of a mother having her baby at home, but also by women having the opportunity to share and explain their change-of-plan experiences without people smacking their hands to their mouths in horror, or exclaiming that they were 'lucky'.

If informed exchanges were more usual, the perceived dangers would get cut down to size and there'd be a fuller opportunity for women to make informed decisions. There is no such thing as a watertight plan. That said, if you are a healthy woman with a well-grown baby and a straightforward, normal pregnancy, the probability of serious problems is sufficiently low and safety sufficiently high for home birth to be a reasonable, positive, valid choice.

Before labour

Certain medical conditions in late pregnancy, in particular preeclampsia, obstetric cholestasis and rising blood pressure, mean there are substantially increased health risks for you and your baby, and it will be recommended that you have your baby in hospital. Other situations requiring careful medical management and where it may be advisable for your baby to be born sooner rather than later can include repeated bleeds, recurring incidences of slow foetal movements, a persistent stalling of foetal growth or broken waters revealing concerning levels of meconium.

Low iron, gestational diabetes (GD) and group B strep may also be red flags in terms of home birth guidelines. But whether you stay at home or not remains your choice and your hospital's duty of care. If, after examining the evidence, you're not persuaded of the risks of staying at home or the benefits of being in hospital, explain this to your midwives and make a plan that feels right for you.

If you are told your iron count is low, get clear on your readings and, if medically necessary, craft a plan to correct it by eating an iron-rich diet and taking iron tablets with orange juice. In just a couple of weeks, levels can be back to normal. Equally, if GD is being controlled by diet, and your overall health is good, talk to your midwife. An automatic abandoning of a home birth plan could be unnecessary.

Be aware that a single rise in blood pressure isn't a de facto hazard in late pregnancy. It's blood pressure that continues to rise that rings serious alarm bells. If you suffer with 'white coat' syndrome and feel a worrying blood pressure reading might not be accurate, have it checked in a chemist or buy your own cuff to be sure.

Apart from in extreme emergencies, there should always be a chance to examine written evidence (research needs to be up to date) on the reason a switch of care to hospital is being suggested and have an open discussion with both a midwife and a member of your obstetric team, remembering that hospital policies are recommendations, not the law.

Dr Rachel Reed, on her blog midwifethinking, has this to say about risk:

Risk is a very personal concept and different women will consider different risks to be significant to them.

Everything we do in life involves risk. So when considering whether to do X or Y there is no 'risk free' option. All women can do is choose the option with the risks they are most willing to take. However, in order to make a decision women need adequate information about the risks involved in each option.

Waters breaking

If you are experiencing a healthy pregnancy, pre-labour rupture of membranes is more likely to affect a home birth plan than a last-minute health issue. So it's imperative to forward-gather a good understanding of the risks and benefits of induction as compared to waiting and have an informed decision ready to hand should this occur.

A big advantage of community care is that you have the opportunity to have a midwife visit you at home to do a few checks. If it's in the middle of the night, and you feel you want to talk to your midwife (you may not), she will ask a few questions and then most likely visit you in the morning – a far more convenient and comfortable plan than having to get out of bed, go to hospital and disrupt a night's sleep.

This, though, is where the benefits end. NHS midwives are working within an integrated healthcare service, and need to abide by their guidelines. It's therefore their job to inform you that ruptured membranes mean there is now a small risk of infection, which rises as time passes, and that the recommended course of action will be to induce after 24 hours if labour hasn't started. This is a narrower window than independent midwives routinely advise (the NHS guideline has gone from 96, to 72, to 48 and now 24 hours, despite no change in the evidence).

It is also their job to explain the facts (e.g. your waters continue to replenish); discuss alternative options, like daily monitoring and generally keeping an eye on you and your baby; encourage you to look at the evidence and be fully informed about whichever choice you make; and, in keeping with NICE guidelines, to explain clearly and impartially that the decision over whether to wait or induce is entirely and completely yours.

There is no having to be induced, and it is not legal for midwives to deny you care should you wish to wait. Key to making a plan is knowing that within 48 hours of waters breaking, 90 per cent of women are in labour. On hearing this, some women feel happy to tolerate the relatively low risk of infection within this window, given the very good odds of them going into labour in the same time period.

A degree of self-care is advisable of course. Introduce nothing into the vagina (this includes avoiding all vaginal examinations); regularly change your pad and check that waters are clear and don't smell; take high-strength vitamin C and monitor your temperature every four hours. Research indicates that taking vitamin C supplements throughout pregnancy, and eating six or seven dates a day from 36 weeks of pregnancy, reduces the chances of waters breaking prematurely.

Group B strep

If you are diagnosed as being group B strep positive, you will probably be advised to abandon your plan to birth at home, and to go into hospital within four hours of delivery to be given IV antibiotics. Research this. Look out good information on the subject so that you can make the best decision for yourself and your baby and feel sufficiently resourced to explore different options. One option to consider might be to look into using herbal and nutritional protocols for reducing GBS colonisation. A garlic suppository is a common home-made remedy to control a vaginal infection.

I was GBS positive. I followed Aviva Romm's recommend-ations (home made suppositories, garlic, probiotics) and tested two weeks after completing them and was negative. I was home birthing, but it gave me a sense of agency and confidence in refusing antibiotics had I been transferred.
Emily

Waiting

Your due date will come, and almost certainly your due date will go. In fact there is a strong likelihood that, along with most women, you won't have your baby until some time between 41 and 42 weeks. These days the wait can feel stressful, as with family phoning every day, and midwives often starting to talk about making a 'plan' at the 41-week appointment, it's easy to feel that something is wrong and your body has forgotten what to do. But if your midwife checks are showing you and your baby are well, and nothing is wrong, then your body hasn't forgotten what to do. Your body has grown a whole human being without you even thinking about it, and has an equally autonomous plan for getting the baby out.

Your due date is not a divinely-ordained certainty. It is the rough mid-point of a five-week distribution curve and it is healthy and entirely normal for a term baby to arrive at any point on that line, right up to and including 42 weeks. Even after 42 weeks, the risks of foetal compromise are extremely low (0.16%) and don't become medically significant, according to the American Congress of Obstetricians and Gynaecologists (ACOG), until 43 weeks (0.21%).

Midwife Gail Hart, writing in *Midwifery Today*, says:

Postdates, by itself, is not associated with poor pregnancy outcome. Extreme postdates or postdates in conjunction with poor foetal growth or developmental abnormalities does show an increased risk of stillbirth. But if growth restriction and birth defects are removed, there is no statistical increase in risk until a pregnancy reaches 42 weeks and no significant risk until past 43 weeks. There is a creeping overreaction in dealing with postdates pregnancies. It is true that the stillbirth and foetal distress rates rise more sharply after 43 weeks, but it is also true that less than 10% of babies born at 43 weeks suffer from postmaturity syndrome (over 90% show no signs). We should react to this rise by monitoring postdate pregnancies carefully and inducing if problems arise. But the rise in problems at 43 weeks does not imply a similar risk at 42 and 41 weeks.

Despite these statistics, many women are still led to believe that once they are overdue, there is a high probability of the placenta deteriorating or abruptly ceasing to function altogether.

But there is no evidence of a direct connection between such developments and a woman being overdue.

Gail Hart again:

The placenta can begin to fail at any point in pregnancy, and part of good prenatal care is monitoring growth and fluid levels so we can act before the baby's reserves are drained. We induce labour—even advise a caesarean without labour—if the baby is in trouble, regardless of due dates. It is obvious that a baby is 'better off out than in' if the placenta can no longer nourish him/her, or if the uterus has become a dangerous place… But induction of labour causes so many problems that it should be a rarity, performed only when the benefits can be proven to outweigh the risks. Induction multiplies the risk of caesarean section, forceps-assisted delivery, shoulder dystocia, haemorrhage, fetal distress and meconium aspiration.

If you find yourself under pressure to accept induction before or by 42 weeks and you are not happy with this, remind your team that the Royal College of Obstetricians and Gynaecologists (RCOG) makes clear that monitoring beyond 42 weeks is an alternative to induction. You can also write a letter to the team manager, so that your choice and your request for support is clearly spelled out.

The fact that your midwife meetings will be in your own community, where it is natural to take control of personal decisions, means there'll be none of the stress that tends to be felt in a hospital setting and you can talk your options through clearly and pragmatically.

Make your midwife aware that your decision is a fully informed one, and if a suggestion is made to talk to a consultant about your reasons for declining induction, remember it is your choice whether you wish to attend. So long as you understand the risks and your choice is informed, you have no obligation to justify your decision.

To bolster patience and empower your body's ability to birth unaided further, beware trading an induction plan for what may appear to be more benign methods of eviction. A forced labour is a forced labour: doing a sweep is just a different form of induction, for example. Even alternative methods, like reflexology or acupuncture, will be bypassing your baby's independent cue for labour to begin.

Getting things going in a 'gentle' way can seem a logical way to avert chemical induction, but if the baby is in the wrong position and not ready when that nudge comes, you're more likely to lose a couple of nights' sleep due to cramping and unproductive contractions than initiate progress. A sensuous clary sage massage; a nightly candlelit bath; a treatment to provide some relaxing you-time; a good daily walk or a hands-and knees wash of your kitchen floor – oh and sex… these are the things that'll help your body to become soft, receptive and ready.

Service arrangements

Sadly, it's not uncommon for women who have planned a home birth to be told that their community midwife team isn't at full capacity and that there may not be a midwife available when she goes into labour. Some interrogation of this curiously flippant flaw in the service will be undertaken in the next chapter. But as regards it presenting a fork in the road, here's my advice: don't let it be.

Though full respect needs paying to the hard work and often tireless dedication of midwives in the UK, the way you would like your baby to arrive in the world should not be at the mercy of NHS resources. Your trust has an obligation to provide maternity care and, as AIMS explains on its website, when you decide to stay at home to have your baby, both the midwife's duty of care (set out in the NMC Circular 8-2006) and government policy clearly sets out a woman's right to choose a home birth.

Around 37 weeks is the most common time for telling women this, because from this time onwards women often cannot face confrontation, and as a result the majority will accept what they are told and change their booking. But according to AIMS, women who are determined to give birth at home, and who make it absolutely clear (preferably in writing) that they have no intention of going into hospital, are 'somehow' provided with a midwife. 'To do otherwise, would leave the trust in an indefensible position were a disaster to occur as a result of their failure to provide a midwife.'

If a message is left on your phone, or a midwife explains this situation at one of your final antenatal appointments, take action and clearly restate that you are requesting and expecting their care in labour. Follow it up with a letter (a template can be found on the AIMS website). Copies should be sent to the head of midwifery, your named consultant if you have one, the chief executive of the Trust and AIMS.

During labour

According to latest research, 45 per cent of first-time mothers planning a home birth end up transferring to hospital (12 per cent of second-time mothers). Not surprisingly, this statistic is discouraging for many women, causing them to think they are better served by the assumed certainties of hospital care. Without a breakdown and analysis of this figure, imagination steps in with any number of wild and frightening images and the decision about where to give birth gets made on unfounded conjecture.

As well as taking a careful look at the reasons for and manner of transfer, it's important to note that there are no hospitals in the UK with a normal birth rate of 55 per cent. This is significant. Also, of 1,000 babies born at home, 997 will be born without serious medical problems. If women having their babies at home have the greatest chance of giving birth by themselves of *anywhere*, without recourse to anaesthesia, chemical drips or other interventions, what does this tell us?

When to move

The first thing to know is that the majority of women who get moved to hospital from home do so in non-urgent circumstances due to slow progress of labour, or because they are requesting medical pain relief. In other words, extra support feels like a good idea. The mother may take a shower, someone may make some tea, bags are gathered and the move is made, either by ambulance or, if preferred, car.

Clinical issues requiring transfer are less likely. The midwife's observations will have provided her with a good picture of how labour has been unfolding, so any issue will be acted on well in advance of it becoming an emergency, and transfer arranged.

Foetal distress is detected by listening to the baby's heart, generally between contractions. A normal heartrate is between 110 and 150bpm and should vary throughout labour. However, a heartbeat that becomes much faster or slower, or very irregular, would be concerning. If position changes make no difference, your midwife will want to get you into hospital, as this is a sign that the baby is not coping well with labour.

In the second stage, once pushing has begun, it is more normal for the heart rate to respond to contractions and dip. As long as it recovers once the contraction has passed, this is fine. A heart rate that slows after the contraction is over (this is called a late deceleration) is a sign of distress and would also raise the question of transfer.

Another possible sign of foetal distress is evidence of green/brown meconium in the amniotic fluid. If this is accompanied by irregularities of heartbeat, it would be advisable to go to hospital. Your midwife will be trained in all aspects of foetal heart compromise and intermittent monitoring will give her plenty of warning of this.

Shoulder dystocia is where the baby's shoulders don't rotate properly inside and get caught on the pubic bone, impeding the baby's exit. This would be an emergency, but the chances of a true dystocia occurring in a normal, physiological birth, where the mother is upright, kneeling or squatting, are extremely low (0.5%). Virtually all steps for management of shoulder dystocia can be undertaken at home, including changes in maternal position or the birth attendant manually freeing the trapped shoulder or using suprapubic pressure. In such a situation, the mother needs to trust, listen and follow her midwives' instructions, as they will be trained for this eventuality and have a sequence of optimal manoeuvres and positions to work through designed to resolve it. Traditional midwife Ina May Gaskin maintains that getting the mother on her hands and knees is the best position for release. Getting the mother to draw her knees to her chest is another.

First breathing

Remember that a well-grown baby is prepared to cope with labour and birth. Not only will assessment in pregnancy have confirmed that heart and lungs are functioning healthily, but also the mother's body 'packs the baby a picnic' prior to labour, laying down extra stores of glycogen so that good circulation is maintained throughout. All this together, along with checks in labour, means that babies almost always take their first breath without help, with the shift in air pressure as they emerge causing their lungs to inflate automatically, like balloons.

A pause before the baby takes a breath is not the same thing as a baby being compromised at birth. It can even take a couple of minutes for the baby to 'come to' – a bit of residual lung fluid may still need expelling, a rub with a towel provides a bit of extra stimulation, and breathing begins, usually accompanied by a little squawk or cry.

Delayed cord clamping is now routine, and rightly so, as it is nature's backup, continuing to provide the baby with a supply of oxygen for at least 10 minutes. This means that so long as the midwife has sufficient light to see, the cord should be left intact. Babies born at home rarely continue to cry once they are cuddled against their mum's chest, so don't be alarmed if, after saying their first hellos, they fall silent.

The chances of your baby needing a significant amount of help to start breathing after a normal labour and without any previous signs of foetal compromise are very, very small, and in most cases are resolved with some suction or a bag and mask.

Being sure

As incidences of extreme emergency are very rare, the decision to transfer to hospital usually means there is time for discussion and an opportunity for you to get clear and feel satisfied with the reasons for doing so. As you are likely to be familiar with your midwives, and have a trusting relationship, it's likely you will be fully in agreement with the decision. However, if you feel you are being rushed or harassed, or even bullied into moving, it's vital that you talk through any concerns you have, and to make sure that you are completely convinced and agree with the need to move your care to hospital.

Author, NCT teacher and founding member of AIMS Nicky Wesson says of transfer:

When women are left with doubts about its necessity or feel that it was for the benefit of her attendants rather than her or her baby, there can be a lingering sense of fury or frustration. If you do not feel convinced that it is necessary, you can ask the following questions:

- *what is the indication for transfer?*
- *what benefit will it have?*
- *are there any risks involved in that course of action?*

- *what alternative treatments could be tried?*
- *what will happen if nothing is done?*

Long labours: a matter of fact or a self-fulfilling prophecy?

Twenty-five years ago, the transfer rate for first-time mothers was 10%, far lower than it is today, as was the incidence of long, unmanageable labours requiring an epidural. Why so? Our bodies haven't changed, and I cannot believe women now are somehow less equipped to cope. That studies show transfer from home to hospital was far lower in home births assisted by independent midwives, rather than NHS midwives, also raises questions.

Several factors have contributed to the rise in non-emergency transfer and while these remain unacknowledged and unexamined, there's neither a chance of the transfer rate reducing any time soon, nor take-up of home as a birthplace choice increasing.

From a care perspective, more stringent guidelines have certainly impacted on how long labour is 'allowed' to take, and there is now less room for individualised assessment. Women are no longer given the time their body might need to give birth, and momentary deviations from the norm, for example a drop in heart rate due to the mother's position, may trigger greater caution than they once did.

Another factor may be home birth midwives having their 'ward' head on, what obstetrician Michel Odent calls bringing 'the hospital to the home.' The disturbing, conspicuous arrival of midwives and equipment, coupled with a less-than-deft introduction of monitoring and observation, can create a break in flow and focus, impact oxytocin release and contraction strength, and trigger a slow-down in labour.

I definitely think my midwives' failure to attune to where I was caused my labour to stall. I'd been in my bedroom all afternoon, lying, leaning, my eyes shut – totally in my own world. When the midwife arrived she insisted on making eye contact and engaging my attention. She plonked all the bags down right next to me and immediately started scribbling notes. I remember what a distraction her biro was, my attention coming back to the room and what was around me. The next thing I felt was a sense of deadline, of feeling watched. It may have been all in my mind, but when you feel observed like that, you can't help but feel a sense of expectation. Every time a contraction came, she did something, a heart-rate check, or moving a bit of equipment, or writing something up. Up until that point, I'd felt so good – so right and safe in my body, but now I just felt so odd and uncomfortable. I couldn't relax, my contractions spaced apart and a few hours later they called an ambulance.

Debra

The option to let go and feel completely unselfconscious are two top benefits of labouring at home. But if a midwife isn't clear on the importance of this, or how to keep an eye without the mother feeling watched, the mother can feel scrutinised, especially as the midwife has no distractions and may make the mother the sole focus of her attention. A birth pool can easily lead to this situation, with midwives and supporters assembled around it like an audience. Overuse of torches and mirrors can draw the mother further awake, and all too commonly labour stalls, especially in the second stage when the mother's naturally increased awareness may become a cue for chat or active coaching.

To avoid this, talk with your midwives beforehand. Get a

sense of their experience, and how much they understand of the physiological need for privacy and the aid it can be. Have your request for subtle, unobtrusive sensitive care laid out in your birth plan, including quiet unless you wish to speak; no updates or discussion of what can be seen while you are pushing (phrases like, 'That's it, that's it, nearly there' or 'That one was a good one' can create too much pressure); and no managing of your behaviour unless there is a good medical reason or you yourself want something to change and want guidance.

On a more specific note, make sure that you are regularly reminded to go to the toilet, as a full bladder can obstruct progress. Also, if you and your baby are well, but labour has stalled, always try some alone-time before any talk of transfer starts. Have your doula or partner help you to get comfortable, for example supported by pillows on your side in bed, drink a full cup of tepid camomile and honey tea, then put on an eyemask or switch off the lights. You'll still need to breathe through each wave, but the effect of complete privacy can work like a miracle. Shifts in position can also help, as well as your preferred comfort measures.

A final reason for an overlong and unmanageable labour can be what we've already covered in a previous chapter – women themselves not knowing what to expect. When it's your first baby, it's easy to want something to happen – to call round your midwife and go into gear, as if somehow that will mean progress and bring your baby closer. It won't. If you aren't in the second room – active labour – and your midwife and doula arrive before things are really progressing, birth can end up feeling way too long. Not actually long, but feeling like it, because the clock started ticking too soon.

If the stage gets set (birth pools inflated, positions taken, candles lit) when you are still building to birth, and are therefore very aware, things can become even more protracted – much as they would if someone sat by your bed, watching you fall asleep. To minimise the chance of transfer for so unnecessary a reason, practise patience and draw on your reserves appropriately. Conserve energy and stamina by distracting yourself and being as self-reliant as possible.

Giving birth without a midwife

Sometimes a baby will arrive before the midwife has got to your house. The most likely reason is that labour is swifter than expected, taking the mother and her birth partner by surprise, or else a midwife is called on time, but for some reason gets delayed.

Either way, it's a good idea to have talked through the possibility, so that you're clear on what to do. This is not so much because the baby needs help – a baby born quickly, without disturbance, is generally very well, as is the mother. It's so that you and those with you can move through the experience calmly.

There's no need for partners to rush about or raise their voice and no one should panic or force the mother to do things against her will. At all costs the mother must be protected from stimulation, and the flow of oxytocin – the key to a safe birth – maintained.

Informing a woman who's pushing that the midwife can't make it will 'wake' her up; involving her in decision-making can create a sudden uprush of adrenaline. So to maximise safety, it's important that the behaviour of those surrounding the mother remains composed and that calls or any obvious decision-making happen out of her earshot.

If it becomes obvious that a baby will very soon be born, make sure the mother is in a safe position, for example lying on her side or leaning forward with soft towels beneath her, and let nature take its course. Babies are designed to birth themselves so do nothing, stay very quiet and trust that both mother and baby know exactly what they are doing. Given there's no choice, do your best to relax and remember that babies were born without medical experts present for thousands of years and that the midwife, or ambulance if you've called one, will soon be there.

Once the baby is born, be ready with a towel and give the baby a little rub if necessary. Let the mother 'find' her child herself. She will probably take a few moments taking it all in, and place a hand on her baby's tummy. Though there'll be a great sense of relief and emotion, avoid creating a sense of rush, or any attempt to arrange mother and baby unless the mother seems to want help.

Once the mother has taken her child onto her chest, wrap them both in a few warm towels or blankets and turn the heating up. If the placenta comes soon after, before the midwife or ambulance crew, just leave it where it is, and don't attempt to cut the cord.

Malposition

Sometimes labour is just long, for no other reason than the baby is in a difficult position. A baby positioned with its back to the mother's back (rather than its back against her stomach) isn't able to apply even, deepening pressure on the cervix (the head rocks off and on due to less room), meaning progress can be slow. Backache is common in this situation as well as contraction pain feeling sharp and jabby, and as a result it's easy for energy to run low and dejection to set in.

A mother in this situation may feel like giving up on her home birth plan and heading into hospital. But in most cases, babies do eventually turn, at which point progress can accelerate, so it's worth trying a few things first to see if the situation changes.

Comfort-wise, huge relief can be gained by holding a hot water bottle in place on the lower back, and pressing it hard when a contraction comes. Very strong thumb pressure, either side of the spine, and just above the knicker line, can have a similar effect, and a warm bath, with the added distraction of a shower on the sacrum when a contraction comes, can all keep a mother going until she turns a corner.

Positions that 'spin' the baby will also help, like:

- kneeling on a sofa and, when the contraction comes, resting both hands on the floor (try through 3–5 contractions)
- deep alternate lunging
- side-lying, with the top leg dangling over the side of the bed when the contraction comes
- rocking hips/pelvis with a shawl or rebozo. Your partner can sling the back wall of your pelvis if you are standing, your bump if you are on all fours. They wrap the cloth ends round their wrists, and 'sift' the cloth to create a ripple through the pelvis.

All of these measures can relieve tension and help your baby to turn. A soothing trick that I've found works well is to lie the mother on her side (supported by pillows) and to take hold of her top leg, by the foot and ankle for example. When a contraction comes, press the knee into the chest, and back again, in and back, levering the leg until the contraction completes.

Tightness in the hips (sometimes a symptom of a brow-presenting baby) can be relieved by vigorous bouncing or figure-of-eighting the hips on a birth ball. Placing a foot on the third step of the staircase and lunging deeply can also create extra space and allow babies to shift.

If pain and slow progress persist and, as doula Penny Simkin says, 'labour starts to feel like suffering,' a move to hospital for medical pain relief can be a positive step. If things are advancing, just slowly, and you need a chance to rest, an epidural may take you from 'blown off course' to 'back on track', so long as you are able to lie on your side and have the chance to sleep.

My first daughter was back to back. I had a lot of back pain, but I coped well for many hours, by moving and humming and making noise. I then got into the birth pool and fell asleep in between contractions and active labour slowed down. The midwives said I should get out of the pool and walk up and down the stairs. They gave me an 'ultimatum'. If I dilated to 8cm in two hours (I think I was at 4cm) then I could stay at home. I squatted, sat on the birth ball, went up and down stairs and was fully dilated after two hours. The waters did not break and I declined them breaking them. They said to start pushing if I felt any urge at all to bear down, so I did. The waters broke and there was a deceleration in the heart rate. I was tired but felt that things were going right and although they called an ambulance I said I wanted to stay home as I felt I was on the home stretch. I said to my partner I wanted to stay home, but he thought it was best to do what the midwives said. At that point I felt a bit lonely and regretted that we had not had a doula or an independent midwife.

I was determined to have a normal birth and once in hospital I kneeled on the bed and held on to the headboard, as that felt right. They said I had to be on my back, but I ignored them. They said if I didn't push her out on the next push, they would perform an episiotomy, so I pushed with all my might and my daughter was born. They put her on the resuscitaire, but I heard her crying and said that I wanted them to give her to me, which they did. It was exactly 30 minutes from the waters breaking to birth; 10 minutes waiting for the ambulance; 10 minutes transfer; 5 minutes to hospital bed and 5 minutes being hooked up and giving birth. Looking back after nearly six years it feels sadder than it felt then. Back then, I felt quite proud for managing with their conditions. I still am eternally grateful I was at home when I was at home.

Regine

After the birth

A postpartum haemorrhage is less likely to happen at home than in hospital. A worrying level of bleeding after birth would be defined as 500ml or above, though in many countries it is 1 litre. The best way to judge what is too much, is any amount of bleeding that leaves you feeling faint or unwell. The two main causes of bleeding are a bad tear or an atonic uterus, where the uterus fails to contract after the delivery. Your midwife will have the necessary drugs to stop bleeding, usually a syntometrine injection, but if she remains concerned she will arrange for you to be transferred to hospital. A complicated tear that the midwife deems would be better sutured in a medical environment would also mean you might be transferred after your baby is born.

Another reason for transfer after the baby is born is a retained placenta. If you are given enough time and the right conditions to birth your placenta naturally (privacy, peace and quiet, and an unhurried chance to meet your baby undisturbed), there should be no problem with the third stage. Explain clearly in a meeting beforehand that you wish the atmosphere and environment post-birth to remain the same as it was during labour – for lights to remain low or off, talk kept to a minimum and, most importantly, for there to be no sense of waiting or expectation (gloved midwives, obviously watching, waiting and asking 'Can you feel anything yet?' can create a surprising amount of stage fright, even in your own sitting room).

Have your preferences for as much privacy (your midwife of course needs to keep an eye on you, but this should be unobtrusive) and calm as possible laid out in your birth plan. If the placenta doesn't come of its own accord, the midwife will recommend an injection of syntocinon or syntometrine, and if the placenta remains retained after that, you will need to be transferred to hospital to have it removed. This situation is more common than you'd think, but could become less so if there was greater understanding of the basics of postpartum physiology and respect for what mother and baby most need. Research this thoroughly and make ready. It can feel a dreadful shame to labour smoothly and give birth at home, only to be lifted from your cosy nest at the very last when, with appropriate low-profile care, it could have been avoided.

I had a very positive home birth with my first son which involved transfer. The birth itself was straightforward, a 10-hour labour, which started with my waters slowly leaking. My son was born into a pool with no other pain relief, in my sitting room, and I caught him myself. After 40 minutes of my placenta not appearing, the midwives were concerned by my blood loss (800ml) and suggested the injection in my thigh to encourage my womb to contract and release it.

This worked well and my placenta obligingly appeared! Sadly, however, as a possible side-effect of the jab, my blood pressure spiked in response. I was then transferred, though not in any panic (I popped on a wash of towels with the ambulance parked outside as I felt fine) and was monitored in hospital after this for a few days.

I was not worried by the transfer, I felt fine in myself, strong and mentally 'with it', and I trusted the midwives, who had left me to labour as I wished during the day – being utterly unobtrusive and nothing but encouraging and calm.

My only negative experiences were in hospital, where I absolutely hated being stitched and breathing gas and air (WAY worse than the birth!) and things were not communicated to me, so I was often left alone not knowing what would be happening next or when.

We are now 28 weeks with our second child and excitedly preparing for a second home birth at which we hope our 2.5 year old son will be present. It will be with the same team of midwives as the first birth and they have discussed how we can try to avoid the same situation reoccurring. Our first experience has only served to highlight how positive, calm and relaxed our first birth felt compared to feeling so out of control and lonely in hospital.

Sophie

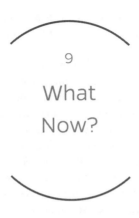

9

What Now?

Having a baby at home makes sense. It is a safe and sustainable choice, it brings health and wellbeing benefits for mother and baby and it gives women a high chance of having a satisfying experience.

In his book *Evidence-Based Care for Normal Labour and Birth*, professor of midwifery Dr Denis Walsh points to there being a 'canon of reassuring literature about the safety of home birth' with new studies confirming the advantages all the time: fewer caesarean sections, fewer assisted vaginal births, lower rates of postpartum haemorrhage, less need for neonatal resuscitation, and fewer birth injuries in the home birth groups than in matched hospital groups.

Though hospital remains an appropriate setting for women in need of specialist care, he writes:

Olsen and Jewells' Cochrane review of 2006 concluded the change to planned hospital birth for low-risk pregnant women in many countries during this century was not supported by good evidence. Planned hospital birth may even increase unnecessary interventions and complications without any benefit for low-risk women.

Personal accounts confirming how birth at home offers an extremely rewarding emotional experience pile up pretty high too. Ask a selection of women who've had their babies at home, and the reports are overwhelmingly consistent. Mothers say they feel strong, free, safe and deeply fulfilled.

And there are further upsides. A personalised birth service at home is cheaper than care received on an obstetric ward, and that's not including the sum saved by the reduced necessity for caesareans, medical interventions and postnatal care on a ward. The caseload model of care commonly used when mothers are supported at home brings mothers and midwives into equal partnership. Birth has its best chance of unfolding normally and babies reap the rewards – immediate opportunity for contact and bonding with their parents, the perfect circumstances for triggering natural immunity and an optimal foundation for first breastfeeding.

The benefits of birth at home are as deep as they are wide.

Yet only 2.1 per cent of the pregnant population opt for it. Despite the medical establishment's open acknowledgment of the advantages of home birth a clinical setting is what most women continue to choose, including the conveyor-belt care that's likely to accompany it.

Though the trend is confusing, the reason for it is simple. Pregnant women and the maternity system are caught in a catch-22. Since 2005, despite greater institutional focus on women's choice and midwife-led support, the normal birth rate has continued to decrease. Women *know* that homogenised hospital care isn't giving them what they need. But the generational lack of confidence that's resulted from women expecting birth to be long, hard and horrible has created a disempowered sense of no alternative; that making do and hoping for the best is the only realistic choice on offer.

It's like the old Jewish joke: 'Two elderly women are at a mountain resort, and one of them says, "Boy, the food at this place is really terrible." The other one says, "Yeah, I know; and such small portions."'

Low confidence means that there's little demand for the kind of quality of care that brings confidence – a learned helplessness that's further fed by media fearmongering and uninformed public negativity.

When women are canvassed for what they actually want from maternity care, over and again they say the same thing: personalised, woman-centred, continuous care that helps them to feel safe, relaxed, respected and at the centre of their experience.

Who wouldn't want these things? The daft bit is that it is already possible! These feelings. This care. THAT kind of experience. All you have to do is join the dots, make the connection and book a midwife to look after you at home.

It was my doula who told me to book in with my local community team. I never thought about home birth to be honest, I was fully expecting to have my baby in hospital, as was my husband. On the day, I had a fairly long build-up period – all night, all morning, all through the next afternoon – strong, testing regular contractions that never really changed – there was no sense of progress, or it being labour proper. Luckily for me, I now had that midwife visit to draw on. She dropped by, reassured me that all was fine, and told me to get comfortable. It helped me cope and relax. That evening, everything ramped up big time and now there was no doubt I was in labour. The midwife came again, took one look at me and said,

'Fantastic, you're doing brilliantly… do you want to move to hospital to have your baby or shall we stay here in your bedroom?' I'm not sure I even answered her, but I think she got the message. My husband was a bit shocked when the midwife went downstairs and explained the plan, but when he questioned it, she replied, 'So do you want me to tell you it's going badly?' Then she told him to go and pour himself a glass of wine. My little girl was born a couple of hours later. It was the most amazing experience of my whole life.

Lucy

A new mood

The good news is that we are waking up. For too long, choices about where and how babies are born have been drawn from a jumble of conclusions.

Women are now increasingly aware that giving birth on a hospital bed, with an unknown midwife, is just the current culture-specific way of having a baby. 'Birth by the batchload' as a mother in my active birth class called it.

According to Nicky Wesson, author of *Home Birth*:

Couples are feeling less comfortable about suppressing the very intuitive feeling that birth should take place in privacy and security and more curious to know how birth might be when it's free of inhibition and tension.

In my own childbirth preparation class, second and third-time mothers are jumping at the chance to explore another way; to do things differently and have their babies at home, many having had their fingers burnt first time. And where first-time mothers used to switch off at the suggestion of birth at home, questions are now asked. Many are first surprised, then excited, to learn that, contrary to what they'd pictured, there is a more intimate and bespoke way to experience this precious life event. Not everyone is open to the idea of course, but those less confident about exploring different possibilities are encouraged and carried by those more sure.

Mothers return to share their experience of giving birth at home, excited and incredulous about what they have felt, and the room comes alive – curiosity firing up and spreading from one to the other, with the result that, regularly, at least half of the class arrange to meet a midwife for an open discussion about the possibility of birth at home.

It's early days of course, but there is evidence of similar surges of interest elsewhere in the country: in Dorchester and Poole in Dorset; Bridgend in Wales; Datchet and Windsor in Berkshire – communities where strong chains of local confidence are growing.

I once heard about a government-funded local project aimed at promoting home birth in Doncaster. Initially interest was low and take-up minimal. But then one mother, on one street, on one estate, had a fantastic experience giving birth at home. She told her pregnant neighbour, who followed suit and took advantage of midwife support in her own home, and had an equally positive time. Word began to spread quickly – it was a close community, and each mother's lived experience spoke for itself. Demand for home birth soared.

Imagine this on a grander scale. Word-of-mouth is a powerful driver, and already responsible for a buzz of positive exchanges between mothers online. While the mainstream media is light years behind the real story, preferring to exaggerate dangers and foment mummy-wars tension, grassroots organisations like the Positive Birth Movement and tellmeagoodbirthstory.com are quietly spreading first-hand news about the ways women shape their births and help themselves.

There are some astonishing pay-offs to information-sharing as opposed to informing-giving – and as a result of it, expectations around birth are rising.

Peak passivity seems to have been reached. A post-feminist mood is drawing women away from a set-up that rests on a fair bit of helplessness and obedience and leading them instead towards a new kind of consumer-think – to taking control of and responsibility for their birth experiences.

Previous trust that a few 11th-hour NCT classes can adequately prepare you for birth is on the wane. Women are ripping up the rule book and giving themselves new proactive permission, making each other, as well as online hubs fizzing with feedback and personal experience, their guide – much as they would a price-comparison site.

More will and must follow as the exclusion of mothers from their central role in the birth process amounts to social control of their bodies, a situation conspicuously and unacceptably at odds with the rest of life. New feminist debate points to the important connection between the domination of nature and the domination of women – that babies being 'delivered' and routine medical management of birth rests unequivocally on the notion that the female pregnant body is a container to be emptied.

Complete equality should surely include women having full and authentic control of their reproductive lives, and the autonomous experience of giving birth under one's own steam, without it being authorised, modified or managed by a third party, is a clear route to that.

I was about six months into my pregnancy when it dawned on me that a hospital setting couldn't give me what I needed. I didn't want to be a procedure. I wanted to be a person. I didn't want an environment I'd need to back away from in labour, I wanted a space I could move into and relax in. And of course that was my home.

Jenny

I remember trying to write my birth plan and having this knot of unease in my tummy. It was so stressful trying to foresee what unknowns I might hit in hospital – all the emotional and practical adjustments I was going have to make. It all felt so irrelevant. So I started thinking about what did feel relevant. And that was comfort and control. I realised I'd have lots of both in my own home – without needing to make provision for them.

Melanie

The service

When a person wants to learn how to do something, they find someone who's done it and copy them. Public objectives can be met by modelling in the same way. If birth at home is to become standard practice, we need examples to imitate. It's to areas with a flourishing home birth service that we should turn.

The average rate of home birth across the country is currently around 2%. But in Sussex and South Dorset it has reached 9%, and in parts of Gloucestershire, Berkshire and Wales, home birth has also succeeded in hitting the 10% mark at times.

In 2009, the home birth rate took a dip. From what had been a steadily rising trend, it dropped and plateaued at 2.3% and in the last year, has dropped further to 2.1%. The RCM pointed to midwife shortages as the cause – explaining that it wasn't home birth demand that had declined, but the availability of dependable midwife home support. This currently remains the case but it's important to know that where NHS Trusts have kept women's choice a priority and policy efforts have been made to sustain and integrate community teams into the overall service, dedicated home birth teams have developed and become beacons of positive practice. Virtuous cycles establish: the more reliable the service, the greater the demand; the greater the demand, the stronger the service.

If this were the case countrywide – if all mothers had a guaranteed local midwife team to rely on – it's estimated that the home birth rate would rise to 10%. This is exactly what happened in South Dorset. Dorchester's 'Cygnet' team is a group of midwives entirely dedicated to supporting women at home and since their launch in 2015, the local home birth rate has increased from 2% to 10%.

So how could that trend be rolled out, and real choice become a mass-scale reality? *Better Births*, the most recent government maternity review, found that women wanted a more personalised, joined-up service and identified the case-loading model of care, whereby women are looked after by one midwife or a small team from the start right through to their birth, as a way to provide this.

It also supported new models of care, for example by ensuring that tariff-based NHS funding supports the choices women make, and by making it easier for groups of midwives to set up their own NHS-funded midwifery services. Surveyed midwives who worked on such teams reported a positive experience. One respondent wrote:

We have a very high home birth rate and are all very confident as a team in providing this service. We promote it and support women's choice and make it the norm when telling women their choices for place of birth. We explain that it is all part of our service and that we are very experienced and confident in supporting women birthing at home.

Partners are advised about our skills and drills training and reassured that we would not offer this service if it was in any way dangerous. Because we are supportive and confident, we give the women and their partners the confidence to have a home birth. It works really well I can tell you, and it is something that our team of 12 midwives in a rural seting are very proud of.

The review expressed concerns about the feasibility of universal case-loading, and some practical suggestions were put forward to address them, for example good rotation of midwives, ring-fencing time for midwives working in case-load teams, so that they weren't diverted to other services, as well as capping case-load numbers to manageable levels.

The first meeting

A reliable midwife service is the central mechanism for giving the greatest number of women the greatest chance of having a baby at home. But it's actually a very simple lever that gets everything moving and a mother thinking. The first meeting. Imagine a newly pregnant woman having the following exchange with her midwife:

Midwife: *Right, that's all your checks, you seem very healthy and your baby is growing beautifully. I now need to give you some information so that you can think about your choices. So firstly... giving birth is very safe for you and your baby, wherever you choose to have your baby. Whichever setting, hospital, midwife-led unit or home, the chance of an entirely normal healthy outcome is very, very high. Go and check out the Birthplace Study and the NICE guidelines – I'll give you the links – and then you can see for yourself and show your partner.*

You can choose to give birth at home, in a midwife-led unit or in an obstretric unit. But you should know that as you are a healthy woman, with a healthy pregnancy, the latest evidence shows that an ordinary medical ward will increase your chances of having interventions and a caesarean. So you might want to look into the other options.

Mother: *That's really interesting. I didn't know any of that... even so, I wouldn't have a baby at home first time. Maybe for my second baby, but first time, there are too many unknowns.*

Midwife: *It's true there is slightly more risk for first-time mothers – 9.3 adverse perinatal outcome events per 1,000 planned home births compared with 5.3 per 1,000 births for births planned in obstetric units – but the risk is still extremely small and needs weighing against the many advantages, for example there being much less chance of an emergency delivery, or an episiotomy. Also remember that we are midwives and as fully trained to take care of you at home as we would be on a ward. We have the exact same safety equipment that there'd be on a midwife-led unit, and we're experienced at spotting any issues well in advance.*

Mother: *Ah, OK, I didn't know that – I just assumed there was a lot more danger, that there are more risks – I thought staying at home would be kind of like winging it a bit.*

Midwife: *Far from it. Not only are safety measures all in place, but also by the time you are term, we'll have a really good picture of your and your baby's health and if you are low risk, you have a very high chance of having a completely straightforward labour. Labour is a completely normal, healthy function of the female body – ask a couple of friends who had positive birth experiences, ask what they read, and do a bit of research. Your body is designed to give birth and your baby completely equipped to cope.*

Mother: *Oh I never thought of it like that, it always looks so fraught on the telly, like there's an emergency every five minutes.*

Midwife: *Yes well, that's telly for you – it's not real. Birth can be a wonderful, positive experience – you can be in charge of it and influence how it unfolds just by setting things up well, by giving your body what it needs to labour. For example, being free to move, and use gravity so that the baby is helped to move down… and making sure you have a calm, quiet, private environment to help the birth hormones flow.*

The thing is, it's not about hospital birth versus home birth. When you've got a midwife booked to come to your home, it's not fixed in that way. It's about keeping your options open. You get to know us, we come and do your appointments at home, and when things get going, one of us will come round and see how you are doing. From there, it's up to you.

An awareness-raising exchange of this nature works wonders on a mother's confidence. It's a prime opportunity to get clear on the facts, and yet according to a survey conducted by the RCM, only 52% of midwives think mothers receive adequate information about giving birth at home.

Other findings in the survey are a clue to why. For starters, only 58% of midwives surveyed said their areas provided a full home birth service all of the time, so it's not surprising that there's hesitance when it comes to promoting it.

Then there's the question of midwife confidence. The survey revealed that a third of midwives receive no home birth training in their initial placement at all, and that there was a strong feeling that further training and education were necessary about physiological birth, the needs of 'healthy, normal women', as well as a greater understanding of why women should consider home birth as a viable option.

There's a simple solution to this. One single adjustment to midwife training would increase confidence a hundred-fold and have requests for home birth soaring: a compulsory requirement for student midwives to attend 10 home births to qualify. Marsden Wagner, perinatologist and one-time Director of Women's and Children's Health for the World Health Organization, said the reason birth has become so dehumanised is because 'fish can't see the water they swim in':

> *Birth attendants, be they doctors, midwives or nurses, who have experienced only hospital-based, high-interventionist, medicalised birth cannot see the profound effect their interventions are having on birth. These hospital birth attendants have no idea what a birth looks like without all these interventions, a birth which is not dehumanised.*

So imagine the opposite scenario – how *humanised* birth would become if birth attendants were guaranteed to observe totally normal birth during their studies. Wouldn't that make sense – for them to see for themselves the astonishing efficiency of labour when women are undisturbed and supported in their own environment?

The effect would revolutionise the way we view childbirth today. Dr Amali Lokugamage, obstetrician and author of *The Heart in the Womb*, found her thinking was transformed in just this way, simply by stepping away from the ward framework she'd been working in for 20 years, where in her words, she knew 'most everything', and giving birth to her own baby at home:

It enhanced my understanding of the humanistic side to labour and delivery. It made me aware of the profound influence of my baby communicating to me and me communicating with my baby.

In comfortable surroundings – your home – the body can unfold itself. Most women, not all, but the majority of women can give birth by themselves as part of their health rather than as a part of disease. When it happened to me, I almost felt as if my baby had said, 'give me the right environment, and I will do it.'

Alignment

We are, as Michel Odent says, at a turning point. There are now more caesarean sections, inductions and surgical interventions performed than ever before; increased postnatal stress and depression as a result of traumatic birth; widespread reduced newborn immunity resulting from increased rates of complicated delivery; the lowest breastfeeding rates in the world and maternity care protocols being ever more governed and shaped by litigation, fear and hospital insurance policies.

Birth is in crisis – but it's a low point that's caused a stir of the right elementary particles to begin to make progress. It's now not so much why home birth matters, as why on earth it hasn't mattered – why we've allowed ignorant, groundless bias to prevail and home birth's dizzyingly beautiful benefits to be brushed aside. With it comes less fear, more faith, and a healthy, hopeful prototype of birth for mothers to rediscover. Watch this space. Five years from now, everyone will know someone having a baby at home.

Further Reading

Books

Home Birth: A Practical Guide, Nicky Wesson, Pinter & Martin, 2006

The Homebirth Handbook, Annie Francis, Vermilion, 2016

The Father's Home Birth Handbook, Leah Hazard, Pinter & Martin, 2011

Birth Reborn: What Childbirth Should Be, Michel Odent, 1994

Birth and Breastfeeding, Michel Odent, Clairview Books, 2007

The Positive Birth Book, Milli Hill, Pinter & Martin, 2017

Why Human Rights in Childbirth Matter, Rebecca Schiller, Pinter & Martin, 2016

Why Doulas Matter, Maddie McMahon, Pinter & Martin, 2015

The New Pregnancy and Childbirth, Sheila Kitzinger, Dorling Kindersley, 2011

New Active Birth, Janet Balaskas, Thorsons, 1990

Ina May's Guide to Childbirth, Ina May Gaskin, Vermilion, 2008

Gentle Birth, Gentle Mothering, Sarah Buckley, Celestial Arts, 2013

The Heart in the Womb, Amali Lokugamage, Docamali, 2011

Do Birth, Caroline Flint, The Do Book Co, 2013

Home Births – Stories to Inspire and Inform, Abigail Cairns, Lonely Scribe, 2006

For reference

www.homebirth.org.uk

www.midwifethinking.com

www.sarawickham.com

www.evidencebasedbirth.com

www.aims.org.uk

www.birthrights.org.uk

www.birthchoiceuk.com

The Birthplace Study: www.npeu.ox.ac.uk/birthplace

Intrapartum Care for Healthy Women and Babies: www.nice. org.uk/guidance/cg190

Nursing & Midwifery Council circular 8-2006: www. homebirth.org.uk/nmc.pdf

NHS England National Maternity Review: www.england.nhs. uk/mat-transformation/mat-review

Thoughts on Homebirth Transfer by Mary Esther Molloy: midwiferytoday.com/mt-articles/thoughts-homebirth-transfer/

A Timely Birth by Gail Hart: midwiferytoday.com/mt-articles/a-timely-birth/

Support

www.tellmeagoodbirthstory.com

www.positivebirthmovement.org

www.doula.org.uk
www.imuk.org.uk
www.neighbourhoodmidwives.org.uk
www.onetoonemidwives.org

Preparation

www.yogabirth.org
www.activebirthcentre.com
www.thedaisyfoundation.com
www.birthlight.co.uk
www.birthpoolinabox.co.uk
www.madeinwater.co.uk
www.hypnobirthingworks.co.uk
www.kghypnobirthing.com

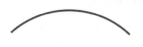

Index